Building a
Research Career

Date Due	Date Due	Date Due	Date Due

This book should be returned on or before the last date shown above. It should be   ested by the library. Fines are ch

Building a Research Career

CHRISTY L. LUDLOW, PhD
RAYMOND D. KENT, PhD

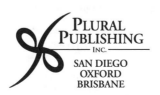

PLURAL
PUBLISHING
INC.

SAN DIEGO
OXFORD
BRISBANE

PLURAL PUBLISHING
INC.

FSC
Mixed Sources
Product group from well-managed
forests and other controlled sources

5521 Ruffin Road
San Diego, CA 92123

e-mail: info@pluralpublishing.com
Web site: http://www.pluralpublishing.com

49 Bath Street
Abingdon, Oxfordshire OX14 1EA
United Kingdom

Cert no. SW-COC-002283
www.fsc.org

Library of Congress Cataloging-in-Publication Data

Ludlow, Christy L.
  Building a research career / Christy L. Ludlow and Raymond Kent.
       p. ; cm.
  Includes bibliographical references and index.
  ISBN-13: 978-1-59756-227-0 (alk. paper)
  ISBN-10: 1-59756-227-0 (alk. paper)
  1. Research—Vocational guidance. 2. Scientists—Vocational guidance. I. Kent,
Raymond D. II. Title.
  [DNLM: 1. Career Choice. 2. Science. 3. Research Personnel. 4. Research.
5. Vocational Guidance. Q 147 L945b 2010]
  Q180.A1L77 2010
  001.4023—dc22
                                                                        2010020946

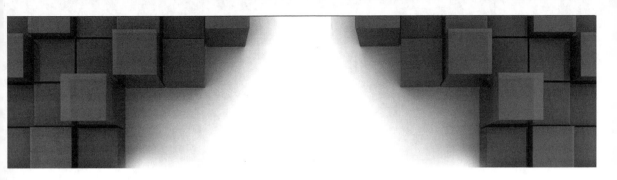

Contents

Preface

This book was written with the goal in mind of including important information we would have liked to have known when we first completed our research training but had to spend several years acquiring. In addition, many things about research training have changed over the last three decades, and the needs of people entering a research career today are somewhat different than they were even a few years ago. New entrants should now expect to have a mentor who will be conscientious about guiding their students and postdoctoral fellows through the long process of building a research career. But, even with such expert help, scientists must chart their own course, and this book is a navigation aid. Science has become more of a team effort; no longer can a scientist work in isolation and be successful. Interpersonal skills are now essential to success. This book explores ways in which an individual scientist can be part of a larger collaborative effort without losing identity and focus.

Competition always has been an aspect of research and credit comes most to the team that publishes significant new findings first. The explosion of new knowledge and the need to remain current have added new challenges and working in teams can be very effective for meeting those challenges, therefore, making collaboration more essential. The pressures from universities and other institutions to obtain external funding from government agencies or private sources has become greater, particularly in stressed economic times, and the importance of external funding to obtaining tenure has increased at many universities.

At the same time, regulations governing research and scientific integrity have increased; and oversight and scrutiny have exploded in all areas of science, but particularly in the clinical research realm. It is imperative for investigators to be aware of these regulations and the accompanying demands on accountability. Although all of these changes have resulted in greater pressure on scientists, the rewards of a scientific career also have become greater. Technology transfer, patents, and commercialization are now part of the scientist's world. In addition, the range and variety of careers in science have increased to include government, commercial, business, and educational, as well as scientific writing for the layman about science. Clinical research has changed considerably. No longer does a physician run a small study on a group of patients; all such trials now must be registered and the data posted on government Web sites before they are published in scientific journals.

Our intent is to introduce the new investigator to the explicit and not so explicit expectations of a research career. The purpose of this book is somewhat different from *Making the Right Moves: A Practical Guide to Scientific Management for Postdocs and New Faculty*, which is focused on bench scientists in biomedical research (Bonetta, 2006a). The focus of this book is directed more to the individual scientist who may also be a clinician, a physician, dentist, pharmacist, psychologist, nurse, or specialist in allied health who may not have been trained foremost as a basic scientist but wants to enter a career in research or combine it with their specific discipline. On the other hand, this is more of a training and reference book in contrast to the very personal book, *So You Want to Be a Scientist?* (Schwartzkroin, 2009), which addresses many aspects of being a scientist in basic research in an academic setting.

We have come from different environments in our careers and have combined to bring both perspectives to this book. Ray Kent has spent most of his career in academia working on basic research in speech science, while educating both speech scientists and speech-language pathologists, chairing a department, running a productive laboratory, and publishing research as well as writing seminal works in the field. Christy Ludlow was at the National Institutes of Health first as a grants and contract administrator for 10 years before becoming an intramural principal investigator in clinical research and combining both animal and clinical research while training postdoctoral fellows, and recently moving her laboratory to academia. We have brought different viewpoints to this book in the hope that it will help those interested in a career in research meet the demands and joys of the exciting challenges ahead.

Finally, there is a no more exciting career than one in research. Although challenging, the deep satisfaction that comes from formulating and testing ideas, making new discoveries, finding answers, and solving problems cannot be overstated. Our hope is that this book and some if its advice will help make the entry and path through a career in research more enjoyable and rewarding.

Christy L. Ludlow, PhD
James Madison University, Harrisonburg, Virginia
Raymond D. Kent, PhD
University of Wisconsin-Madison, Madison, Wisconsin

In memory of
Sadanand Singh, PhD
A kind and gentle friend
who maintained a peaceful optimism
no matter what life threw at him.

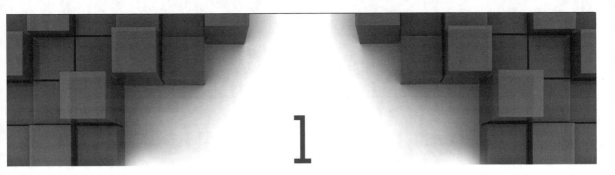

Career Stages in Research and Characteristics of a Successful Scientist

INTRODUCTION

The different stages of a career in research include: initial research training at the doctoral (PhD) level, postdoctoral training, tenure-track junior scientist or assistant professor, tenured associate professor or principal investigator at a research institute, and full professor or senior investigator at a research institute (Figure 1–1). For clinical investigators, the different phases for a research career can be intertwined with the required phases for clinical training and credentialing including: medical school or other professional training; internship and residency or clinical credentialing; board certification or specialty training; followed by clinical practice in academia.

The focus of this chapter is on the research stages in a career and what it takes to be a good scientist. It is important to understand these stages to plan a career and for a clinical investigator to decide how to integrate research and clinical training. For example, whether to do the clinical credentialing before or after the research doctorate must be considered, unless candidates are in a joint PhD-MD training program where the two are interleaved or a PharmD/PhD program.

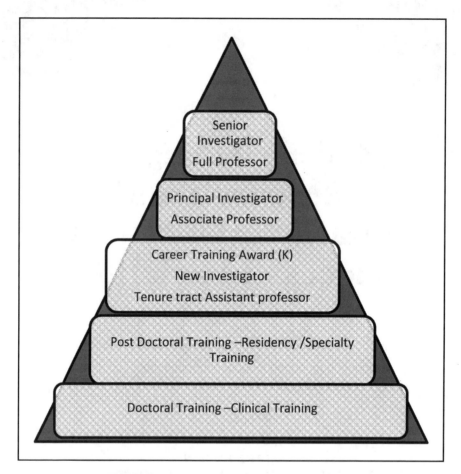

FIGURE 1–1. Stages in a research career.

THE STAGES OF A CAREER IN SCIENCE

Selecting a Doctoral Program

The PhD is the entry level for a research career and the required credential. Although the PhD is the entry level for a research career, there are large differences in the training offered by different universities while studying for a PhD. Several aspects should be considered when applying for a doctoral program: the candidate's area of interest, the mentor, the institution, and the candidate's research goals. All usually are addressed in making the decision regarding where to apply (Figure 1-2).

Most important is the mentor. For the first 5 to 10 years after completing a PhD degree, the first question often asked is, "Who did you study with?" Thus, the mentor's reputation determines the types of postdoctoral positions

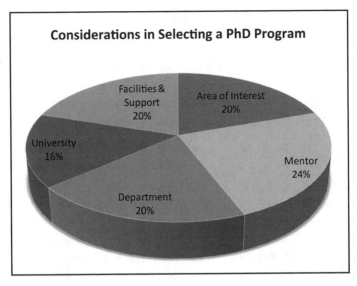

FIGURE 1–2. Relative importance of different aspects when selecting a PhD program.

a candidate will be considered for as well as tenure track faculty positions. Chapter 3 addresses how to search the literature for citations of a person's work. To evaluate a mentor it is good to use Web of Science, EigenFactor, or other resources (see Chapter 4) to identify the numbers of citations of a person's research in an area of interest. After discounting techniques papers and review articles that often are cited but may not have contributed original research, the frequency of citation of an individual's research articles can identify the impact that a person has had in their field. If a person's work is frequently cited then others are aware of their research and they might be a good mentor.

Also, it is important to determine if a potential mentor has research funding. Doing a search of the Research Portfolio Online Reporting Tool (RePORT, http://projectreporter.nih.gov/reporter.cfm) of research grants supported by the National Institutes of Health will identify grants held by a prospective mentor. Similarly, grants from the National Science Foundation, the government agency supporting basic research, can be searched at http://www.nsf.gov/awardsearch/. Someone with more than one grant is less likely to lose all of their grant support at one time and have to close their lab. It should be possible to determine the length of funding for a current research grant. If a potential mentor has a newly funded 5-year grant, then the likelihood of a stable research environment for the duration of doctoral training, which is usually around 5 years, is high.

Equally important to the reputation of a mentor is mentoring style. Others who have worked with that person can be most informative about how easy a person is to work with, mentoring style, and how supportive the mentor is to trainees. To some degree, it will depend on the style of the mentor the candidate is most suited for. Some mentors use the "sink or swim" approach, that is, they leave students to solve their problems, organize their exposures, and learn from others; if the student does, fine, they are very supportive. However, this type of mentor is not beneficial if a candidate does not have a good idea of what he or she wants to learn and is not already self-directed. Other mentors are very detail-orientated and want to make certain students won't fail; for some candidates, this can be intrusive; for others, this is welcome. Therefore, candidates need to consider what type of mentor they will do best with, how self-directed they are, and whether they already have their goals well laid out and the amount of guidance they think they need before deciding what type of mentor is best suited to them. Asking others for their opinion of what kind of mentor to choose can be helpful; we are not always the best judge of what we need in our research training. Previous mentees can be located by looking at previous publications of the mentor. Normally, doctoral students and postdoctoral students are the first authors on publications and the mentor is the last author, that is, the senior author.

Also important is to consider if other faculty are available in case the choice of a mentor does not work out. Sometimes mentors leave for another institution and the student cannot follow, become ill, move to an administrative position, or the mentor and student do not get along. There should be others that the candidate could work with on the same faculty.

Of next importance is the reputation of the department, the institution, and the other faculty in the department. Some research-intensive universities or institutions (referred to as RI Institutions) have large numbers of laboratories and clinical research programs that are well funded by NIH grants to academic faculty. Often shared research facilities are available such as electron microscopy, protein or drug screening, sequencing facilities, functional imaging, and central animal care and surgery facilities, which serve large groups of investigators. Such universities support doctoral students through research grants that allow them to work in faculty laboratories as the basis for doctoral training. The only way to learn research is through working in a research setting. Such universities often have medical schools and can support students working in both laboratories and large clinical research programs. A listing of RI universities can be obtained from the Web site of the Association of American Universities (AAU) (http://www.aau.edu/about/article.aspx?id=5476). It lists 62 leading public and private research universities in the United States and Canada. Universities are invited to membership in the AAU based on the quality of their academic research and scholarship and undergraduate, graduate, and professional education in a number of fields. Member institutions are recognized as outstanding based on the excellence of their research and education programs.

Some institutions have training grants with slots for pre-and postdoctoral students from the federal funding agencies such as the National Institutes of

Health, the biomedical research funding agency of the United States Government. A list of research training grants (T32) from the National Institutes of Health for any particular institution can be retrieved by doing a RePORT search (http://projectreporter.nih.gov/reporter.cfm). Searching for a training grant in a content area can identify institutions that might have openings in a particular field.

Third is the type of training and the tools the candidate needs for the type of research they are planning. For example, if a candidate is interested in neuroimaging research and the program has no access to functional or structural magnetic resonance imaging, it would not be a good choice.

Guidelines for Selecting a Doctoral Program

1. Decide on what you want to learn, what area of research you are interested in.

2. Identify experts in that area and determine who the leaders are in the field.

3. From among those leaders, find mentors in your area of interest whom you can feel comfortable with. Often, you want to contact them at a meeting; or email them ahead of time and arrange to meet with them. Then if you are further interested, arrange to visit them, their laboratory, and their institution.

4. From among the mentors you identify, determine their programs/departments, and other faculties to narrow down to about a half dozen programs that will be able to provide you with training in the skills you want.

5. Learn which programs have openings, and the type of funding they have available.

6. Find out what each program expects of their doctoral students. Are they supported to work on research full time or are they expected to teach or be involved in clinical training at the same time.

7. Speak to other doctoral students, present and past. What do they like or not like about the program.

8. Find out how long it normally takes to get a doctorate in that department —if it is too short, 3 years or less, there may not be enough time to learn the skills you need. You should aim to complete your degree in about 5 years. It is important to have adequate time to publish two or three studies before you graduate so that you can be competitive when applying for postdoctoral training positions. Ask how many doctorates has the program awarded and how long the average person took to complete it full time.

9. Apply to several programs. You may find that you like or dislike a program once you have visited it.

10. What is the track record of the department and Institution for helping doctoral students write and obtain pre- and postdoctoral research grants from foundations, the National Institutes of Health, and the National Science Foundation?

Postdoctoral Training

Postdoctoral training is almost essential to prepare for a faculty position in the sciences. On arriving at a university, to get started quickly and effectively, a new faculty member's research program should be well formulated in advance. By doing a postdoctoral fellowship, fellows should have time to design their research program ahead of time. A new faculty member should know how to get their lab set up, and already have the conceptual framework developed for their first grant application. At the postdoctoral level, the area of training should complement doctoral training by adding an additional area of expertise. Postdoctoral fellows can learn another discipline or set of techniques that will allow them to develop a unique research program.

Here the postdoctoral mentor and his or her area of expertise are of the greatest importance to deciding on where to go for a postdoctoral fellowship (Figure 1-3). The mentor for postdoctoral training will be important in helping fellows compete and prepare for a faculty position.

During postdoctoral training, fellows usually will work with the mentor in the laboratory, although other postdoctoral fellows and graduate students likely will be in the same laboratory. Candidates should visit before deciding

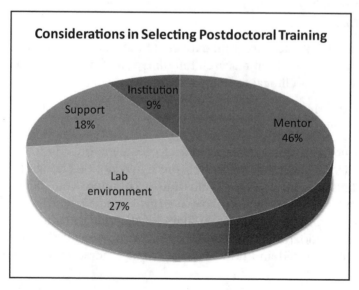

FIGURE 1–3. Relative importance of different aspects when selecting a postdoctoral position.

on a mentor and see the atmosphere in the laboratory. They need to learn how available the mentor is or whether they will need to depend on others in the laboratory for training because the mentor often is out of town. This is not an unusual situation but fellows need to be assured that the necessary support is available.

Fellows should be exposed to different perspectives on science in their field during doctoral and postdoctoral training. For example, different scientists may have varying opinions on the validity of a new method, the significance of a new area of science, and the importance of a new technology. Gathering information on others' opinions always serves to identify "sensitive" areas to avoid, particularly in grant applications. A mentor should help a postdoctoral fellow in moving to greater independence from doing a few well-designed studies to developing an individual program of research.

A postdoctoral position should be at least 2 years and preferably 3 years. The first year is spent learning the new techniques; the second year involves designing and conducting studies, and the third year writing papers and interviewing for a faculty position. A candidate should always speak to others who have trained with a potential mentor to see if he or she is supportive of fellows. Some scientists tend to direct fellows too closely and treat them like research assistants rather than helping them move toward greater independence.

Becoming a New Investigator

After postdoctoral training, junior investigators will move to start their own laboratories either as tenure tract faculty members in academia or as new investigators in a research institution. A new investigator may need to consider other opportunities besides academia particularly in times of financial difficulties for academic institutions when new faculty openings may be few. Tenure track faculty positions also are becoming scarce and very competitive in some fields, and in some cases people choose to do a second postdoctoral fellowship until they can find a good position.

Other opportunities are to be a scientist in a medical school department although such positions are usually "soft" money positions, that is, funding is usually provided for the first 3 years as a start-up package with the expectation that salary will be supported primarily by research grants after the initial start-up period. The advantage is that there will not be a large teaching load other than a few lectures to residents, and less of the other demands such as serving on committees. Such scientists are expected to provide research training to medical students and residents in their laboratories for short periods of time, usually less than a year and often 3 to 6 months. Scientists in these positions also are expected to help junior medical faculty design their research and develop grant proposals.

As a new investigator at an institution, either as a faculty member or a scientist in a medical school, the "start-up" funds are essential for setting up a new lab. Planning on the timing of when to purchase and set up the laboratory also is important. A new investigator needs to gather pilot data as soon as possible, so they may want to stagger setting up different components over the first 2 to 3 years. Later, as one area is established, a combination of "safe" and more "risky" innovative projects may be beneficial (Figure 1–4). Starting with the safe project is advisable but it must be significant as well; venturing into more risky innovative ground-breaking projects should be emphasized only when the new investigator is more secure in their position and funding. Chapter 10 deals with strategies for succeeding in academia.

The National Institutes of Health and many foundations emphasize support for new investigators, by recognizing new investigator grant applicants and giving them funding at higher percentile scores. Because this occurs only at the beginning of a career, new investigators need to use this preference wisely and take great care to submit the best application possible. Review committees have memories and one bad first impression can have lasting con-

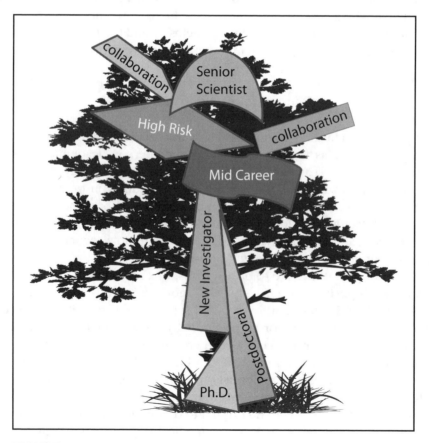

FIGURE 1–4. Mixtures of risk and collaboration at different stages in a Research Career.

sequences. New and old investigators should leave time to have others look at their best drafts and expect to revise their application many times. Often, there is the tendency to assume members of the review committee are experts in the same area and do not need the rationale spelled out for experiments or procedures.

As investigators develop their research, they need to stagger an array of funding sources such as the National Institutes of Health (NIH) and the National Science Foundation. Staggered funding is important to maintain a laboratory, as even a brief lapse in support can result in the loss of trained personnel and essential resources. If a Veterans Administration (VA) Medical Center is nearby, gaining an appointment at a VA will allow an investigator to apply for VA research funding for a project relevant to veterans health. In addition, the investigator's own institution usually has starter grants of small amounts to pay for supplies and a part-time research assistant. Alternatively, a start-up package may include support for a couple of graduate assistants to work in a new investigator's lab. Foundations also support new researchers focused in a particular disease area, and provide low levels of support to enable a new scientist to start a project and gather the pilot data essential for an NIH grant proposal.

Mid-Career Scientists and Collaboration

"Team science" is now expected as it is recognized that several different areas of expertise may be required on a project and no one person can be adequately sophisticated in all areas. The fit of several investigators on a project must be justified but a team of co-principal investigators (PIs) can often be very competitive in the grant system. Collaboration can be particularly good for a new investigator to develop expertise from a senior scientist who is a leader in the field. However, this must be done sparingly as the tenure track investigator must demonstrate that they can work independently and have their own area of investigation. Often, others see collaborations as a way to broaden their base of funding and welcome the opportunity to work with others, particularly once tenure has been granted. However, there are pitfalls when things fall through the cracks or one person does not do their part of the work, holding up the overall project. In approaching a collaboration, it is best to spell out in writing each person's responsibilities and time lines so that everyone knows what they are committing to.

Creating a Mix of Safe and Risky Science

Many scientists have more than one focus in their laboratory so that if one area of research gets bogged down by a difficult problem, progress can be made in another area. Often giving postdoctoral fellows a combination of a "safe" and a "risky" project allows them the opportunity to do something groundbreaking but not lose all of their research if the risky project runs into difficulty. Therefore, a scientist may have two areas of research that pertain to the same issue but are different aspects, for example, a study of the factors involved the development of a brain region and another set of studies aimed at how injury to that brain region during development can produce plastic changes in neighboring regions with training.

At different stages in a research career, combinations or safe and risky projects will change in distribution, with risky projects coming later (see Figure 1-4). At the initial stage in a career, a young scientist must first demonstrate his or her independence whereas later that scientist is better able to develop collaborations once they have become recognized as an expert in their own right. The reasons for collaborations will change from initially wanting to learn from experts, to later being able to expand knowledge into another area of research related to a scientist's ongoing program of research (see Figure 1-4). Generally, in the initial stages of a career, both risk and collaborations are kept to a minimum. Once an investigator is more secure he or she can develop new areas that may have greater risk but have increased potential for greater payoff and impact. Some scientists maintain both safe and risky projects, with appropriate allocation of time and resources. The safe projects ensure continued publications and result-oriented progress reports, whereas the risky projects open the possibility of innovative research with high impact. The recent focus by the National Institutes of Health on innovative research with a high impact has emphasized this aspect of a research support.

Senior Investigators

As a scientist grows and matures reaching the stage of full professor and/or senior investigator, they become a leader in their field. Often, they are called on to write review articles, serve as editors of journals in their area of expertise, be on symposium panels and give keynote addresses at scientific meetings. Their role in promoting their scientific discipline and enhancing research support through advocacy in scientific societies becomes important to the health of the scientific discipline. Collaboration is enhanced as senior scientists are called on by others because of their expertise and knowledge in their field.

Scientist Emeritus

With retirement, many scientists continue to be productive. Their institutions award them Scientist Emeritus allowing them to use the library, may provide office space and access to other facilities while they play supportive roles in their scientific discipline.

CHARACTERISTICS OF A SUCCESSFUL SCIENTIST

Being a scientist is an exhilarating, although often challenging, career. Many of the attributes below are mentioned in a recent book on life as a scientist (Schwartz-kroin, 2009). To be successful requires many of the following attributes.

Love of Science and Curiosity

A scientist needs to love the discovery process and enjoy learning as a lifelong endeavor. Science can call for a great deal of work and dedication, and without enjoying the processes of discovery and learning, a person usually will not stay with it for a career.

Discipline and Focus

To be successful, a scientist must be able to focus and have a great deal of self-discipline through long hours of hard work and frequent obstacles. Getting an experiment correct requires taking care of many minute details, solving the instrumentation, validating methods, and perseverance to ensure success. Persons who only like to dabble in multiple things often will not stay with something long enough to make significant advances.

Flexible Thinking

Frequently an experiment will not reach the expected result; the scientist must be able to quickly absorb and rethink their ideas to adapt to changes either in their own results or in the findings of others. A frequent trap is to begin to believe so firmly in a hypothesis that when the data of others' results do not support it, a scientist cannot quickly absorb the results and refine his or her own thinking.

Tolerance for Failure and Criticism

Not every experiment works or reaches a successful result. Publishing manuscripts and submitting for research grants means that the scientist may repeatedly undergo criticism with intermittent successes. Using that criticism to revise and resubmit allows the scientist to improve their work, benefit from the input, and grow as a scientist.

Leadership Skills

To run a lab and be a principal investigator requires working with others, encouraging them, giving direction, and making the long hours of work rewarding and meaningful. Helping doctoral students and postdoctoral fellows through the process of completing a research study, encouraging them, and helping them cope with failure is required. A principal investigator also must be able to take charge, and have boundless determination and enthusiasm to lead and inspire others.

Organizational Skills

As a scientist progresses through the different stages of a research career they often have to take on increasing responsibilities: managing a research program, training students, teaching courses, writing grants, writing manuscripts, reviewing grants and reviewing manuscripts, organizing and running scientific meetings, chairing committees, budgeting funds, and keeping track of expenditures are essential. As a result, multitasking, delegating, and organizational skills are important. Having a good staff is paramount and a lab manager becomes essential as the laboratory grows.

Networking Skills

Being a successful scientist is being a community member, sharing ideas, helping others, doing favors, and returning favors. Introducing your mentees to others and helping them make contact also is important. Getting to know others in the field so that they are aware of you and your work is essential for recruiting doctoral and postdoctoral fellows and placing your mentees in good departments once they leave.

Of course, scientists vary in their personality and personal and work habits as much as any group. Some are extroverts, others are introverts, but both are highly successful. The characteristics listed above are skills that should be honed to achieve maximum success.

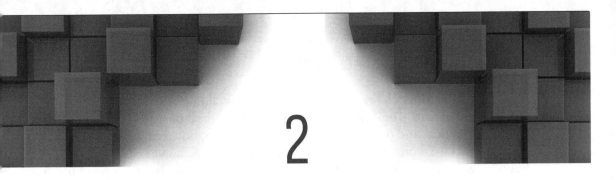

2

Designing Research

*D*esigning research is one of the most important skills for a successful research career. The successful scientist has a research program with overall goals, which then contain specific projects sequenced to achieve specific aims within those overall goals. Because funding mechanisms vary from 1 to 2 years for initial grants from foundations or institutional starter grants to the 3- to 5-year periods for full grants from the federal government, the successful scientist develops a research program to encompass a range of short- and long term goals that will have a significant impact on scientific knowledge or patient care.

This chapter highlights some considerations in designing research; it is not a comprehensive review. In particular, some of the trade-offs to be considered are emphasized.

TYPES OF RESEARCH

The purpose of research is to gain new knowledge for either increased understanding of how organisms function or clinically relevant research to prevent, diagnose, or treat diseases and disorders. This chapter examines the different types of new knowledge that can be gained through various types of research, including basic, translational, clinical, or discovery research and designs for approaching each type of research.

Basic Research

Basic research is aimed at new knowledge regarding how nature functions. For example, one aim might be to understand how neuronal firing in the basal ganglia modulates brainstem nuclei for maintaining respiratory rhythm control in mammals. The goal is to understand the central nervous system control of respiration, and to increase understanding about how two brain regions may interact to control respiration. Such research is aimed at increased knowledge about the neural control of respiration per se without any need to address human function or how this system is altered in disease (e.g., neurologic disorders such as Parkinson disease). The species selected for study may depend on ease of study, cost, availability, and the level of scientific knowledge already available about the species. For example, the availability of brain atlases on a species for locating particular brain regions for neurophysiologic and anatomic study is important for neuroscientific study. On the other hand, if particular genetic factors are the focus, then the mouse might be a better option because of the availability of knockouts or specific mutations in certain strains bred in the mouse. Finally, as discussed in sections on animal care and use in Chapter 6, efforts must be made to reduce the numbers of animals, refine the procedures that are used to reduce pain and suffering, and use a species that is less sensitive to animal rights groups' concerns. For this reason, although the dog may be a better model for cardiac research given its size, care must be taken to limit the numbers of animals used and to consider other species that are less sensitive such as the pig.

Basic research often is focused on understanding biologic mechanisms in species where the system is relatively simple and allows for reductionist models that can be quantified well but may have limited relevance to human functioning or disorders. For example, studies of brain mechanisms for vocalization in the songbird, and the zebra finch in particular, are relevant for studying brain mechanisms involved in synaptic neuroplasticity at different time points in the development of song learning. The relevance of such research to the development of human speech has been questioned given inherent differences between the mammalian and human brain on the one hand and the avian central nervous systems on the other (Jarvis, 2004).

In recent years, scientists applying to the National Institutes of Health have had to be more concerned with how closely their research addresses clinical concerns in humans due to increased emphasis on translational research by the U.S. Congress. On the other hand, basic research on increased understanding of biologic systems per se is very appropriate for consideration by the National Science Foundation.

Translational Research

Translational research is research on mechanisms that have clinical relevance to disease. The purpose of translational research is not to learn more about biology per se but rather to have an animal model of a disease state from which to either understand the underlying brain abnormalities and/or develop potential new avenues for treatments that may benefit patients.

Animal models of disease may be used to explore new treatment approaches. Injections of 6-hydroxydioamine (6-OHDA), a neurotoxin, will cause necrosis of dopaminergic neurons in the substantia nigra and striatum of the brain in many mammalian species producing a model of Parkinson disease (Schicatano, Peshori, Gopalaswamy, Sahay, & Evinger, 2000). Such models then can be used to develop new treatments. For example, the stimulation of endogenous stem cell production may be studied in these models to test the ability of such cells to provide functional replacement for the lost neural cells (Kruger & Morrison, 2002; Lichtenwalner & Parent, 2006; Nakatomi et al., 2002). The limitation of such a model is that it does not emulate the progressive nature of a neurodegenerative disease. Animals can recover to some degree from 6-OHDA injections; therefore, this model may not be relevant to intervening in patients with a slowly progressive neurodegenerative disease undergoing constant adaptation and increasing neuropathology over time. Alternatively, if a human disorder is due to a protein misfolding, a corresponding animal model, such as a transgenic mouse, can be developed to verify the mechanism involved in the human disease (LaMonte et al., 2002). Furthermore, in animal models of stroke, small interfering RNA (siRNA) can protect the brain from ischemic damage by inhibiting the HIF-1α induced apoptotic pathway at the RNA level in a rat (C. Chen et al., 2009).

Clinical Research

Clinical research is aimed at improving knowledge to prevent, diagnose, assess, cure, or treat diseases in humans. The medical model of research is relevant here (Figure 2–1). Diseases or disorders are considered to have an initial cause that produces an abnormality—an enzyme deficiency or a brain development abnormality such as loss of axonal guidance to the original neural target that may result in a deficit later in life.

The initial cause of a disease or disorder is referred to as the *pathogenesis* and may involve a genetic risk factor coupled with an environmental trigger. Research on the epidemiology of a disease to identify environmental risk factors is aimed at understanding the pathogenesis of that disease. Genetic research on allelic variations that may be associated with the occurrence of a disease also is aimed at pathogenesis, whereas research on viruses that make an individual susceptible to a disease is another example. The long-term goal of research on pathogenesis is to prevent a disease by disrupting or reversing the process of disease development once the disease mechanisms have been identified.

Often, however, the original cause may be far removed from the current abnormality, that is, the symptoms or deficit. For example, a child may have a genetic defect affecting the development of axons and their connections between different brain regions. Now the child is an adolescent and shows evidence of a learning deficit affecting performance in school. The original cause is far removed from the particular cognitive deficits that the child now

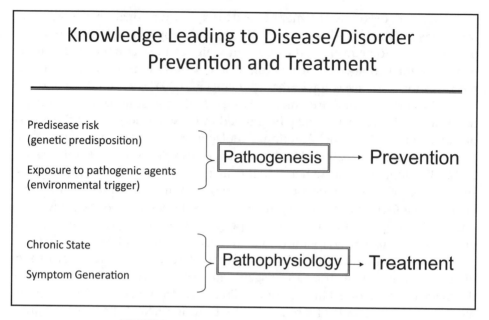

FIGURE 2–1. Translational research aims.

exhibits and it is unlikely that the original pathogenesis can be reversed in adolescence.

In this case, research on the *pathophysiology*, that is, the types of difficulties that are currently contributing to the child's learning deficit, might be addressed in the adolescent child, most likely through specialized training, medications, or both. Studies on the pathophysiology of the disorder are aimed at determining abnormalities that might be contributing to the patient's current difficulties. Such abnormalities are not the cause of the disability but may be a downstream result of the cause. At this point, the focus usually is on the abnormality that contributes to the child's difficulty and how the child may be helped by treating that disability. Another example is when the original pathogenesis was an enzyme deficiency that resulted in cell death for a particular type of neuron. Here the patient's pathophysiology may be secondary to the missing cell types in one brain region (Khan et al., 2005) and stem cell implantation in the region potentially could be aimed at replacing the lost cells with omnipotent stem cells that may differentiate into the types of neurons that normally function in that region (Correia, Anisimov, Li, & Brundin, 2005).

Discovery Science

This is a relatively new approach that tries to identify new methods of treating disease without going through the laborious steps of determining the mechanisms responsible for the pathogenesis and pathophysiology of a disease. Here, the underlying abnormality is unknown but screening is performed in large cohorts of patients to identify differences in protein expression or interstitial RNA that might reflect the result of an underlying abnormality that might be addressed by a pharmacologic or biologic treatment. Once a deficiency is identified, therapy could be used to replace the deficient protein without knowing the original cause of the deficiency (Mathisen, 2003). Thus, the disease could be treated without knowing the pathogenesis of the disorder.

The expectation is that *discovery* science may lead more quickly to new and effective treatments for disease without having to spend decades doing studies to first determine the pathway leading to the development of the disease. However, on the other side, discovery science can be expensive and risky in that a protein abnormality may not be the sole deficit in a disease.

DESIGNING RESEARCH

The Importance of Having a Hypothesis

With the exception of *discovery* research, the importance of a testable hypothesis to a research study cannot be overestimated. Usually, an investigator has formulated a research question; the framing of the hypothesis is the next step as it proposes a specific answer to the research question. The hypothesis allows the investigator to answer the research question by examining the data.

The clinical investigator usually has a hypothesis about whether a particular factor causes a disorder (pathogenesis), or what may be the underlying deficit in a disease (pathophysiology), or which type of treatment might be more effective for a particular disease. A basic scientist may want to study how a respiratory rhythm is generated within a small neuronal network and may hypothesize that some neurons in the circuit have a spontaneous bursting pattern to generate the rhythm.

Having a clear hypothesis and testing it in a controlled research study can ensure some result of the research and the development of new knowledge. Both manuscript reviewers for peer-reviewed journals and reviewers of grant proposals expect a clear hypothesis that can be tested by statistical analysis of the data. The statement of the hypothesis dictates the type of research design, the methods for statistical analysis of the data, and the types of conclusions that can be reached.

It is not essential that the hypothesis be correct, rather that it can clearly be tested by the design and the analysis of the data so that some conclusion can be reached on whether or not the hypothesis is true. This will guarantee that new knowledge can be gained from the research. Without a well-framed hypothesis and the data necessary for testing it, no knowledge can be assured to result from the research.

Because of the need for new knowledge, research that does not test a clear hypothesis often does not receive as high a rating in grant applications or review for publication in many peer-reviewed journals. For this reason, descriptive research often does not receive as high a rating. Although results emanate from descriptive research, without a specific question being addressed, there is no guarantee that the new knowledge gained from descriptive research will have significance. As monies available for funding research by the federal agencies such as the National Institutes of Health and the National Science Foundation always are limited, the *significance* of the new knowledge to be provided by proposed research has paramount importance in grant application reviews. If no clear hypothesis is to be tested, the significance of the research is not guaranteed. This affects the evaluation of *discovery* research, which may have no guarantee of success in identifying a possible defect. If a large number of proteins are being screened, the expectation that a deficiency in protein expression will be identified that will have direct involvement in the pathogenesis or pathophysiology is not guaranteed, making the research high risk and possibly inconclusive.

Framing the Hypothesis

A hypothesis usually is a particular solution to a research question. For example, "the patients receiving treatment X will differ in outcome from patients receiving Y," is a testable hypothesis. This is a *nondirectional hypothesis* in that patients receiving treatment X are not expected to have a greater or a lower outcome score than patients receiving treatment Y. The hypothesis does not suggest that the scores of one patient group will be greater or less than the other group but only that they will only differ in outcome. The probability of a difference by chance alone may be 5% (Neely, Hartman, Forsen, & Wallace, 2003) including two possibilities, either those receiving treatment X may be greater than those receiving treatment Y or those receiving treatment Y may have greater scores than those receiving treatment X by chance alone (Figure 2–2). The two possibilities could each occur with 0.025 probability (Gliner, Morgan, Leech, & Harmon, 2001).

The computation of a test statistic determines whether the value obtained could have occurred by chance alone. If the statistic value obtained would be expected 95% of the time by chance alone, then the null hypothesis of no difference between groups may not be rejected. If the statistic value would be expected by chance alone only 5% of the time, then rejection of the null hypothesis may be acceptable. A 5% chance that the results would have occurred by chance alone often is acceptable. For the entire experiement, the probability of rejecting a hypothesis of no difference between groups by chance alone is usually set at 0.05. That is, if there is more than one test of the same hypothesis within an experiment, then the probability of each of the tests within the experiment will need to be adjusted so that the experimental probability sums to 0.05. Thus, if there are two tests, then the probability to use for each test is 0.025.

Testing the Hypothesis

Two types of errors can occur when testing a hypothesis (Figure 2–3). Type I error is when you falsely reject a null hypothesis when it is true. That is, you decide that the two groups differ when in reality they do not. Usually, you use

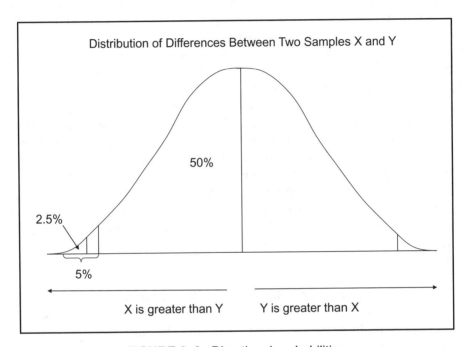

Distribution of Differences Between Two Samples X and Y

50%

2.5%

5%

X is greater than Y   Y is greater than X

FIGURE 2–2. Directional probabilities.

Types of Errors

True Situation	Decision	Decision
No Difference	Reject Null Hypothesis Type I	Fail to Reject Ho
Difference	Reject Null Ho	Fail to Reject Hypothesis Type II

FIGURE 2–3. Errors accepting and rejecting hypotheses.

a 5% percent probability as the criteria for significance—the alpha level—that is, you want to be 95% certain that you are not rejecting the null hypothesis by chance alone. The lower the alpha level you use, the less likely you will find a difference by chance alone and erroneously reject the null hypothesis (a Type I error).

The other type of error is a Type II error when you fail to reject the null hypothesis when it is not true, that is, you fail to find that two populations differ when in reality they do. When there is a high chance of a Type II error, statistical power is low (M. Jones, Gebski, Onslow, & Packman, 2002). Statistical power can be low when the number of subjects studied is too few, and/or the intersubject differences are high. The usual chance that is acceptable for a Type II error to occur is around 20%, that is, you want to be correct 80% of the time when you fail to reject a null hypothesis.

In general, most studies have an independent variable, the experimental factor, and the effect of the experimental factor on dependent variables is being determined. An example is the effect of exposure to a toxin during development in infant rats. The dependent variables are factors that are being measured to determine the effects of the independent variable (the application of the toxin). For example, measures of cognitive development may be used to determine whether exposure to a toxin had a deleterious effect. This is an example of a translational research study conducted in animals.

Dependent Variables and Multiple Comparisons

If the same hypothesis is tested more than once because several dependent variables are measured, then *multiple comparisons* are being conducted of the same hypothesis. This will affect the probability of finding a difference by chance alone. If the probability used in testing the hypothesis desired for the experiment was 5% (i.e., alpha = 0.05), and if the same hypothesis is tested more than once, then the chance of finding a difference by chance alone increases and become greater than 5%. The chance of finding a difference by chance alone can be estimated by multiplying the alpha value by the number of comparisons being used. For example if five variables are being measured yielding five comparisons being conducted to test the same hypothesis, the chance of a Type I error becomes $5 \times 0.05 = 0.25$. To correct for this increased probability of a Type I error, the criterion probability, or alpha, used to reject the null hypothesis must be adjusted, referred to as a Bonferroni correction, by dividing 0.05 by the number of tests of the same hypothesis. In the instance of 5 outcome variables, 0.05 should be divided by five resulting in a Bonferroni corrected criterion alpha level of 0.01. Other methods can be used to correct for multiple comparisons, for example, in neuroimaging where thousands of pixels in the brain are being tested (Ashburner & Friston, 2000).

On the other hand, if the alpha level is being adjusted for multiple comparisons to decrease the chance of erroneously rejecting the null hypothesis when it is true, the chance of a Type II error, that is, not rejecting the hull hypothesis when it is not true also can occur. By correcting for multiple comparisons by using a more stringent alpha level, the chance of a Type II error, of not finding a difference when there is one, can then increase.

The concern with the Bonferroni method of correcting for multiple comparisons is that it is too stringent and could produce a Type II error. That is, by dividing alpha (α) by the number of tests (n) of a hypothesis within an experiment, a Type II error is likely to occur, and a difference could go undetected. This is particularly a concern in fields with large data sets such as epidemiologic and public health research (Levin, 1996). Another alternative is the Holm procedure, which provides for sequential testing of p values by starting with the smallest p value. If it is less than α/n, then move on to the next smallest p value and test whether it is less than $\alpha/(n-1)$, and then continue on in that way until the smallest p value cannot be rejected (Holm, 1979). This method is considered superior for large data sets (Aickin & Gensler, 1996).

Statistical Power

Statistical power is the likelihood of correctly rejecting the null hypothesis when it is not true. A conventional level of acceptable statistical power is 80%, that is, you want to correctly reject the null hypothesis when it is incorrect at least 80% of the time. Statistical power depends on the alpha level you are using when testing a hypothesis, the amount of variance within each of the samples, the degree of difference between the samples, and the number of subjects you are testing in your sample. Care must be taken when identifying the dependent or outcome variables as the number of dependent variables will define the alpha level that you should use.

When many dependent measures are used and the alpha is corrected for multiple comparisons, the probability of being able to detect a significant difference if one actually exists can be decreased and the power of the investigation is lowered. Often, the tendency is to measure many dependent variables in the hopes of finding a factor that was altered by the experimental variable. However, because each time the same hypothesis is tested, the possibility of finding a difference in a dependent variable by chance alone must be adjusted or Bonferroni corrected, and the numbers of subjects required for the study to have 80% power will increase. Usually, an experiment is designed to reduce the chance of a Type II error to 20%, that is, the chance of rejecting the null hypothesis when it is actually incorrect will occur 80% of the time. An example of the difference in the number of subjects required for the same hypothetical experiment with different numbers of comparisons on outcome or dependent variables is shown in Figure 2–4. By increasing the number of outcome variables, the number of subjects required will increase.

The trade-off between the numbers of outcome variables, the probability of a Type I error (set by alpha) and the probability of a Type II error (the power), and the required numbers of subjects per group are all somewhat dependent on the size of the difference in the means of the two groups you

Comparisons in Number of Subjects Needed with Differences in Numbers of Dependent Variables

6 Dependent variables

Number of Groups:2
Within Cell Standard Deviation:3.000
Mean(1):12.000/Mean(2):16.000
ALPHA:0.003
POWER:0.800
Required sample size=19 per group

3 Dependent variables

Number of Groups:2
Within Cell Standard Deviation:3.000
Mean(1):12.000Mean/(2):16.000
ALPHA:0.017
POWER:0.800
Required sample size=14 per group

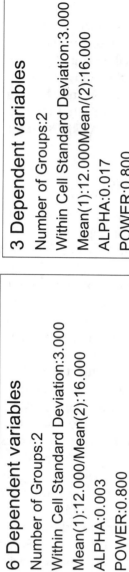

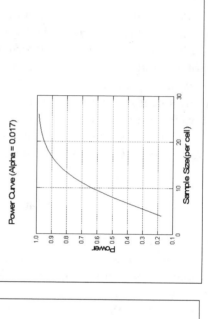

FIGURE 2–4. Changes in subjects required with added dependent variables.

are trying to detect. The size of the difference in the means between the two groups and how it relates to the variance among all the subjects is referred to as the effect size.

Effect Size

The effect size is the amount of change (or difference) in the outcome variable as a result of the experimental variable relative to the overall variance in the outcome variable within the population. Often, the effect size is a much better indication of the significance of the outcome of an experiment than the statistical probability of the result (Gliner, Morgan, & Harmon, 2002b). The trade-off between the numbers of outcome variables, the probability of a Type I error (set by alpha) and the probability of a Type II error (set by the power), and the required numbers of subjects per group are all somewhat dependent on the size of the difference you are trying to detect and how it relates to the variance within the subject groups. In general, the greater the effect size, the higher the power and the smaller the number of subjects that will need to be studied. The greater the mean difference in the dependent variable due to the independent (or experimental) variable relative to the standard deviation, the greater the effect size. The effect size is important when designing a study and determining how many subjects are needed to reach a power of 80%.

Effect size is a metric that is used to compare the results of studies when they have used different statistical methods, different numbers of dependent variables, different sample sizes, there were different variances between subjects within a group, and the amount of difference between groups, which can alter the probability of the obtained result (Imel, Wampold, Miller, & Fleming, 2008). Because experiments often differ in statistical power depending on sample size, the variance, and so on, many investigators prefer reporting of the effect size. In fact, the American Psychological Association (2001) has recommended reporting effect sizes rather than statistical significance.

Depending on the type of statistic that is being used, different measures of the effect size can be computed (Gilner, Morgan, & Harney, 2002a). One measure of effect size is r^2, which indicates the degree of relationship between two or more variables. The r^2 measures the proportion of the variance that can be accounted for by the predictor variable. Therefore, an effect size of $r^2 = 0.5$ indicates that 50% of the variance in one variable can be accounted for by the other variable, which is generally considered a moderate effect, whereas an effect size of 0.3 is small, indicating that the effect can account for only 30% of the variance. In Figure 2-5, the same power and alpha levels are used and the mean difference between the two examples is the same, = 4. However, as the standard deviations increase from 6 to 10, the effect size lowers from 0.6 to 0.4 and the number of subjects required per group to find a significant degree increases from 17 to 45.

Reduced Effect Sizes When Standard Deviation Increases

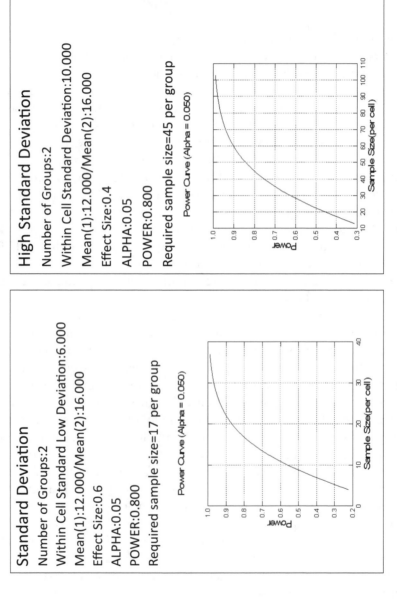

Standard Deviation

Number of Groups:2

Within Cell Standard Low Deviation:6.000

Mean(1):12.000/Mean(2):16.000

Effect Size:0.6

ALPHA:0.05

POWER:0.800

Required sample size=17 per group

High Standard Deviation

Number of Groups:2

Within Cell Standard Deviation:10.000

Mean(1):12.000/Mean(2):16.000

Effect Size:0.4

ALPHA:0.05

POWER:0.800

Required sample size=45 per group

FIGURE 2–5. Changes in effect sizes with differences in standard deviation.

Standardized measures of effects sizes are r^2, Cohen's *d,* and the odds ratio (Cohen, 1992; Gliner et al., 2002a). Cohen's *d,* is the ratio of the difference between the means divided by the standard deviation of the pooled variance of the two samples. In the example in Figure 2-5, the effect size decreased as the standard deviation increased.

The odds ratio is used when the outcome is binary; for example, the numbers of patients in remission at 5 years compared to number with cancer recurrence. For example, if 20 of 48 patients are in remission, the odds ratio of recovery is 20 to 28 or 0.71 to 1, which is low. If another treatment has a recovery rate of 30 out of 48, the odds ratio is 30 to 18 or 1.6 to 1, which is higher. Here, the effect size is the odds of recovery with one treatment over the other. In our example, this would be 1.6 divided by 0.71, which equals 2.25.

Another measure of effect is the confidence interval, that is, the range in values expected 95% of the time. In general, the smaller the confidence interval the better the population parameter is defined, such as the mean of a group. This depends on the standard deviation within a sample. Confidence intervals can be calculated if the sample is normally distributed about the mean, using the values on a Z distribution for probabilities of less than 97.5% and greater than 2.5% to compute a 95% confidence interval. That is, the upper limit will be the mean plus Z times the standard deviation and the lower limit will be the mean minus the Z value times the standard deviation. Therefore, the standard deviation will determine the range of the 95% confidence interval. When the outcomes of multiple factors are being examined using odds ratios, confidence intervals can be used to compare the effects of various factors as illustrated in the following study (Kariv et al., 2006).

When designing a new study, some estimates of the means of each of the groups and the pooled standard deviation are needed to compute the sample size that will be needed. If no published data from the same population are available, then pilot data are needed to demonstrate the mean and standard deviation expected for the research. Many of the statistical packages allow researchers to compute the required sample size based on sample means, standard deviations, the alpha to be used, and the selected statistical power for relatively straightforward types of statistical analyses (e.g., SPSS® and SYS-TAT®). For more elaborate designs, a dedicated program may be used and is often used by biomedical statisticians (nQuery®).

RESEARCH DESIGNS

The medical model for clinical research is aimed at either determining the *pathogenesis* of a disease for the purpose of identifying factors to be manipulated for the prevention or cure of the disease or disorder, or determining the *pathophysiology* for the purpose of intervening after the disease or disorder has occurred for treatment (Figure 2-6).

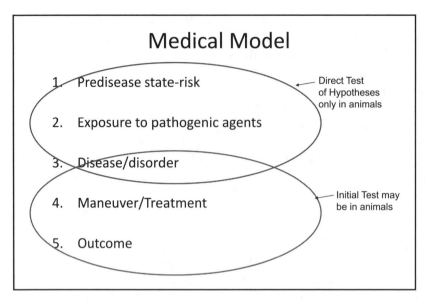

FIGURE 2–6. Medical model for research.

Pathogenesis of Disease

Research on the pathogenesis of disease, and translational research in particular, is aimed at either understanding the development of a disease or disorder by identifying factors involved in the development of a disease or factors that predispose persons to be at risk of developing a disease/disorder. For example, genetic research in large families with a disease initially may identify a linkage site that is associated with the occurrence of a disease or trait. Then, by sequencing a region between markers that confine the region, a particular mutation may be identified. To confirm that the mutation is the cause of the disease or disorder, then an animal strain with the mutation the same as the human mutation must be developed and tested to determine if the same disease or disorder occurs in the animal model.

As a first step, epidemiologic or genetic studies require an accurate identification of persons who have the disease or disorder. For that reason, a very first step in determining the pathophysiology may be the development of an accurate diagnostic test for the disorder. If a biological abnormality is known to occur in all patients affected by the disorder, such as the lack of a particular enzyme, then a *biomarker* for the disease is available and can accurately detect who has the disorder and who does not. Another example would be a biopsy for a specific cell type in tumors. Biomarkers are very useful for future research on the pathogenesis of a disorder as they can be informative regarding the potential mechanisms of disease as well as providing tests for accurately identifying who has a disease. All too often, however, biomarkers are not available and measures of symptoms must be used to identify persons affected by a particular disease/disorder.

Diagnostic Validity

A first step, then, in determining the pathogenesis of a disease or disorder is being able to accurately identify who has the disease or disorder. Prospective studies comparing the new diagnostic technique with the accepted gold standard are required to determine that the diagnostic method is valid (Table 2-1). In many disorders, diagnosis may depend on symptom quantification and a test procedure for identifying who has the disorder and who does not will need to measure symptoms. Research demonstrating the validity and reliability of a diagnostic test may be the first stage in the long process of identifying the pathogenesis of a disorder.

The *sensitivity* of a diagnostic test is the percentage of persons known to have the disorder who are correctly identified as affected. Clearly, only a small proportion of false negatives (persons with the disorder who are missed) is acceptable (Figure 2-7). On the other hand, the diagnostic test also must have *specificity*, that is, identifying only affected persons and not persons who are unaffected (i.e., have few false positives, persons who do not have the disorder but are incorrectly identified as affected). Receiver operator curves (ROC) are used to quantify how accurate a diagnostic test is for identifying cases (Figure 2-8). Tests should have high sensitivity and good specificity. The *x*-axis in ROC is 1-specificity and the *y*-axis is the sensitivity. Tests are accurate with values placement on an ROC curve in the upper left-hand quadrant; in this example test "a" is adequate whereas test "b" is not.

Epidemiologic Research

Often, the first indication of risk factors will come from epidemiologic studies. Once accurate diagnostic tools are available, studies can identify risk factors. For example, case-control studies can compare factors in affected persons or *cases*, with the rate in controls (Figure 2-9). The difficulty with case-control studies that are retrospective is that they may depend on recall and affected persons tend to have biased recall. If risk factors are based on past recall of events, patients are more likely to have considered certain possibilities that may relate to their disease and are more likely to be biased to report a high frequency of a certain type of event in their past than the controls. For this reason, although retrospective studies are easier to do, they often are inaccurate. They can be more accurate if examinations are used to determine the presence of other factors. Such studies often are the first step in identifying relative risk (RR) ratios but must be confirmed through prospective research, which is more costly, particularly if the incidence (the rate of new cases occurring) is low in the population. In a prospective study, two groups are selected based on occurrence of an exposure and then followed to see if the two groups develop certain disorders at different frequencies. Such studies ordinarily can be conducted only in animals.

TABLE 2–1. Levels of Evidence for Determining Diagnostic Validity

Type	Class	Blinded Evaluation	Cohort Size	Design	Comparison Groups	Dx or Outcome Measure	Systematic Application	Measure(s) Used	Sensitivity	Specificity
Diagnostic	I	yes	Broad	Prospective	Control	Gold standard	yes	Systematic tests	yes	yes
Diagnostic	II	yes	Narrow	Prospective	Control	Gold standard	yes	Systematic tests	yes	yes
Diagnostic	II	yes	Broad	Retrospective	Control	Gold standard	yes	Systematic tests	yes	yes
Diagnostic	III	yes	Narrow	Retrospective	Control	Established	yes	Systematic tests	no	no
Diagnostic	IV	no	Narrow	Retrospective	no	no	no	Expert opinion	no	no

2 X 2 Table

Group	Diagnostic test	Attribute measured
Affected cohort	68% identified as affected	Sensitivity= 0.68
Unaffected cohort	12% identified as affected	Specificity=0.88

FIGURE 2–7. Sensitivity and specificity.

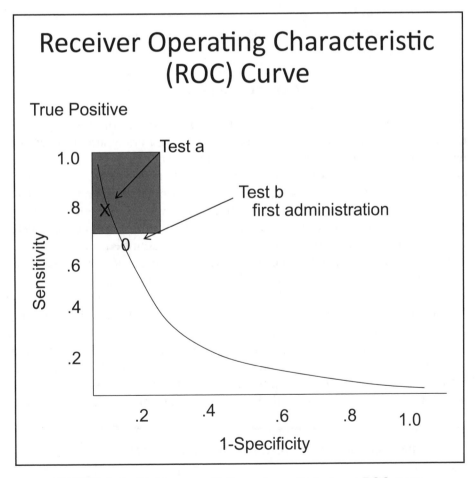

FIGURE 2–8. Plotting sensitivity and specificity in an ROC curve.

Clinical Research to Identify Risk Factors

1. Diagnostic Testing
   - Sensitivity, specificity
   - Receiver operator curves

2. Case-Control Studies (retrospective)
   - Rates of Exposure
     - Relative Risk = proportion of exposed /proportion of unexposed
     - Durations of exposure
3. Prevalence of disorder in different populations

4. Prospective/Longitudinal Studies (prospective)
   - Prevalence after exposure

FIGURE 2–9. Methods for identifying risk factors.

Genetic Research

If a disorder is considered to have a genetic basis, that is, the RR of persons having a disorder is much higher among family members of affected patients than among controls without affected family members, different approaches are used to identify the possible location of a single gene that may be involved in the development of a disorder. Initially, autosomal dominant disorders, where it was likely that only one mutation was involved, were identified by examining for the association between a specific disorder and certain allelic markers. Many of the early family linkage studies identified markers associated with disease occurrence and then, through sequencing within the range identified, could locate the genetic abnormality. Many behavioral disorders are likely more complex, involving multiple genetic modifications and/or genetic and environmental interactions. Here, large whole genome screening is needed, which is more costly.

Once possible risk factors, such as genetic mutations, or environmental exposures, or genetic and environmental interactions, are identified by epidemiologic or genetic studies in humans, only experimental testing in animals can confirm the contribution of these factors for causing a disease or disorder.

Animal Research to Determine the Pathogenesis of Disease

Only animal studies can directly test hypotheses regarding the pathogenesis of a disorder by manipulating genetic risk factors such a genetic mutations or the occurrence of environmental factors such as exposure to toxins or injury. Such animal studies can compare different strains or groups with different genetic mutations before or after exposure to a risk factor. Variation in the mutations or exposure levels can be studied using dose-response curves to determine at what levels of exposure does disease occurrence increase to a significant degree. By being able to manipulate intrinsic or extrinsic factors, the cause of a disease can be experimentally demonstrated using animal studies (Figure 2–10).

Pathophysiology

The purpose of research on the pathophysiology of a disorder is to understand the abnormalities present in the persons with the disorder and to improve treatments for management of the abnormalities in persons with the disorder. This is research aimed at determining what abnormalities may account for the patient's symptoms that, if corrected, might reduce symptoms and hence the degree of disability experienced by persons with the disease or disorder. This may not relate to the pathogenesis, which may be removed in time and in the disease process and may be long-standing.

A hypothetical example might be measuring which muscles have spasms in patients with blepharospasm. Such new understanding then could be used to determine which muscles should be injected with botulinum toxin to reduce involuntary eyelid closing in such patients. This treatment might allow patients to drive a car (a functional outcome) or go out in public without drawing attention to themselves, (a significant improvement in a patient's quality of life).

Pathogenesis-Animal Models of Disease Development

- Genetic risk factors
    - Mutations
    - Allelic variations
- Exposures to environmental agents
    - Dose response curves to identify durations and severity of exposures intervening agents
    - Types of injuries
- Interactions of intrinsic and extrinsic risk factors
    - Do certain risk factors modify the response to environmental exposures

FIGURE 2–10. Animal models for translational research.

TREATMENT STUDIES—THE RESEARCH SEQUENCE
LEADING TO CLINICAL TRIALS

If the pathophysiology of a disease has been identified, then treatment trials can be aimed at addressing the underlying abnormality. Because of the possible adverse effects of a new treatment the first time it is used in humans, to ensure safety, the effects of such treatments usually are examined first in animal studies. Furthermore, if there is a valid animal model of a disease, such studies can also be used to examine how treatment might affect symptoms. This is translational research and the first step in developing new treatments. One difficulty can be the limited predictability of an animal disease model to the human. Sometimes new chemotherapeutic agents for metastatic tumors may reverse tumor growth in animals but have severe side effects or not be effective in humans. Animal trials of new agents often are referred to as preclinical trials and usually are essential before initiating the use of a new chemical or device in humans. The Food and Drug Administration (FDA) regulates all research studies that are first uses of new drugs or first uses of a drug for a particular disorder (application for a new indication) under Investigational New Drug (IND) regulations. Similarly, for devices, new devices first being used in humans are regulated under investigational device exceptions (IDE) that must be applied for from the FDA.

IND/IDE applications need to address potential risks and benefits by reporting results from previous animal studies and early human studies. In an initial Phase I study, the major concern is potential risk. Measures of adverse effects include rate of infection, weight loss, or biological function abnormalities. Serious adverse events are events that cause death, permanent injury, the need for hospitalization, or extended hospital stay. For new chemotherapeutic agents, dose-response curves are used to determine which dosages (e.g., milligrams per kilograms) are most effective and produce fewer side effects. Also of importance are potential benefits: including preclinical animal studies as well as human treatment responses (reduction in symptoms, increased survival, or reduction in tumor size).

Case Series

Case series often involve the first use of a new agent for treatment and are aimed at determining adverse effects and side effects such as nausea and risk associated with first administration. Serious adverse reactions must be reported within a number or days to both the institution, the IRB, and the FDA. These may be unrelated, possibly related, likely related, or related to the treatment, and each instance must be assessed to determine if the research should be stopped, modified, the dosage changed, or the administration altered. An initial case series, often referred to as a Phase 0 clinical trial, involves only a few cases usually where no other treatment has been effective and there is a need to treat the patients to prevent further significant negative impact on the persons involved. No controls are included as there is no concern about the degree of benefit of the treatment at this stage, only the risk involved.

Phase I

This stage also is not involved with determining the degree of benefit; the emphasis again is on risk and adverse effects. A larger series of patients may be involved with a wider range of dosages being studied to determine what may be a safe level for drug administration. Some report of disease or disorder benefits may be included, but because no controls are involved, the emphasis is on the safety aspects of the new treatment.

Phase II

Phase II trials usually involve a control group for comparison with the experimental treatment with some attention being given to both the benefit and the risk associated with the new treatment (Table 2–2). Random assignment may be included to avoid investigator bias, although sample matching also may be used to prevent experimenter bias from interfering with assignment of patients to group. The unconscious tendency to assign patients with a better prognosis to the new treatment can bias a study. Masking or blinding raters who measure the outcomes is essential to ensure independence of the outcome measures from bias. Double blind experiments are used to blind not only the investigators to which group a patient is included in but also the patients. In some trials involving surgery, double-blinding is difficult without a sham surgery; otherwise, patients may become aware about which of the procedures they have received and be biased. Trials involving sham surgeries sometimes show evidence of a placebo effect (Deuschl et al., 2006); in other cases, implantation with stimulation can produce negative effects (C. C. Chen

TABLE 2–2. Design of Random Controlled Clinical Trials

Study Population	Was it well defined, similar characteristics of 2 groups
Randomization	Done beforehand
Blinding	Patients and staff and those doing outcomes
Intervention	What was different between the treatments?
Outcomes	Well-defined, one major variable
Statistical Analysis	Effects of treatment differed, effect size
Funding	Independent from commercial interests

et al., 2006) demonstrating the importance of placebo controlled studies (Horng & Miller, 2007). Usually, a new treatment must be evaluated against the gold standard of treatment for a disease/disorder. After the Helsinki Accord of 2000, untreated placebo groups were considered unethical. If an effective treatment is already known, it is unethical to withhold effective treatment from patients involved in research. Phase II trials generally are small random controlled trials conducted at one center that are aimed at determining the risk-benefit ratio prior to deciding on whether or not to proceed to a full multi-center clinical trial. Such studies often are referred to as feasibility studies and are aimed at determining whether or not a new treatment is more beneficial than the gold standard for a particular patient group.

When experimenters are blinded, a Data Safety and Monitoring Board (DSMB) must be included to review the data at regular intervals. The DSMB should be independent of the research team and the principal investigator and have access to all of the data. The role of the DSMB is to monitor the research for indications of whether a trial should be stopped or altered to protect patient safety. The DSMB must determine if there are: significant increases in adverse events in patients receiving new treatments or particular dosages; differences in the outcomes that would indicate that one patient group is benefiting to a much greater degree than the other and the less effective treatment arm should be stopped; or one patient group is having significant adverse events that would warrant stopping the trial for patient protection.

A Phase II design compares patient groups on their treatment outcomes, such as change scores for an outcome measure of symptoms or disease parameters, and should also include a quality of life measure (Table 2–3).

Phase III

Phase III trials usually involve multiple centers with random assignment and double-blinded controls. That is, neither the patients nor the investigative team know which patients are in the experimental group. Sometimes designs include stratified assignment of different patient groups to treatments to allow for determining whether a treatment is most beneficial for patients with certain characteristics, such as severity, who may have a greater benefit. Such studies require a formalized data management system that is independent from the investigators. In multicenter trials, all of the participating centers must follow the research study design (protocol) using the same procedures and research team training is usually formalized. All of the necessary controls should be addressed to prevent experimenter bias, patient bias, rater bias, and bias due to commercial support (Table 2–2). Here the DSMB plays a significant role and usually reviews the data at regular intervals, such as annually or after a predetermined number of patients have been added to the trial. Phase III trials yield Level 1 evidence and usually several Level I trials showing similar results are required in a premarket application before the FDA will approve a drug for market.

TABLE 2–3. Levels of Evidence for Treatment Trials

Type	Class	Blinded	Groups	Design	Groups Equivalent	Group Assignment	Exclusion/ Inclusion Criteria	Outcome Measure(s) Used	Dropouts Accounted	Cross- overs
Therapeutic	I	yes	Experimental and control	Prospective	At baseline	Randomized	yes	blinded	yes	yes
Therapeutic	II	yes	Experimental and control	Prospective	Matched	No	yes	blinded	yes	yes
Therapeutic	II	yes	Experimental and control	Prospective	Experimental and control	Randomized	yes	blinded	no	no
Therapeutic	III	no	Pre-post measures	Prospective	Patients are own controls	Not random	yes	Independent from treatment	no	no
Therapeutic	IV	no	no	Retrospective	No	No	no	Expert opinion	no	no

35

Quasiexperimental Designs

Sometimes investigators propose designs that are not experimental, such as comparing two treatments within the same patients, referred to as a crossover design, with the order of treatments being given to patients both randomized and counterbalanced. The patients may be blinded to which treatment they are receiving. However, such designs are fraught with bias, the patients will be comparing the two treatments and which treatment they receive first may bias their response to each treatment.

Other designs may be studies where one group receives treatment and the other is on a waiting list; again, this biases patients, those receiving treatment will clearly expect a higher level of benefit over time that those not receiving treatment.

Patient and Clinician Bias

Whenever a new treatment is being compared to a gold standard, care must be taken to ensure that the patients in the study have not previously received the gold standard therapy without benefit as they clearly will have a lower set of expectations for the gold standard treatment. Similarly, clinicians often are biased in their beliefs between the gold standard and the new therapy and questionnaires should be administered beforehand to identify possible clinician bias.

Patient Compliance

No study should be conducted without determining patient compliance as differences in patients in following the treatment regimen can alter the benefits of even the most effective treatment (Coscarelli et al., 2007; Patel, Patadia, Holloway, & Rosen, 2009; Wasserman, Murry, Johnson, & Myers, 2001). If the investigative team does not measure patient compliance, they will not be aware of a major factor that can account for differences in treatment outcomes (Zeller, Schroeder, & Peters, 2008). The problem with patient compliance is the difficulty in quantifying it (Zeller, Taegtmeyer, Martina, Battegay, & Tschudi, 2008). Patients usually want to please the investigator and often inflate their reports of following a treatment regimen. Electronic methods are often more reliable than patient report (Zeller, Ramseier, Teagtmeyer, & Battegay, 2008; Zeller, Schroeder, & Peters, 2007). In any clinical trial, it is important to use measures of patient compliance that are valid and reliable to the same degree as the outcome measures.

QUALITATIVE RESEARCH

Qualitative research comes from the social sciences, including sociology, psychology, and anthropology, as a way of codifying information from inquiry. It can be used as an exploratory step in learning more about a phenomenon prior to developing hypotheses for testing later using quantitative research methods (Charmaz, 2006; Creswell, 1998; Creswell & Plano Clark, 2007). An example might be to learn more about factors that may play a role in introducing a new treatment or service for a disease in a community. Focus groups might be conducted to learn about patients', physicians', and community leaders' concerns and degree of acceptance. The discussion would be transcribed and the responses coded based a system for categorizing responses into different types such as remarks about acceptance, benefits, rejection, beliefs, concerns, cost, burden, and so forth. Software programs can be used to accumulate remarks in different categories and associations between categories; one example of such a software system is NVivo (http://www.qsrinternational.com/products_nvivo.aspx).

Use of qualitative research inquiry has become very important in addressing issues in patient care delivery. The Veterans Administration Quality Enhancement Research Initiative (QUERI) was developed through qualitative methods (Stetler et al., 2006).

When a researcher wants to understand a phenomenon, qualitative research methods can be used to identify important factors that will later need to be systematically measured to develop more rigorous quantitative measures for research. Therefore, qualitative research methods are often a first step. However, qualitative research is very time intensive as it requires careful transcription of responses and the development of a coding system for including as many of the responses as possible. Although a necessary first step, the investment in time and effort is not trivial and must be planned with experts in this arena.

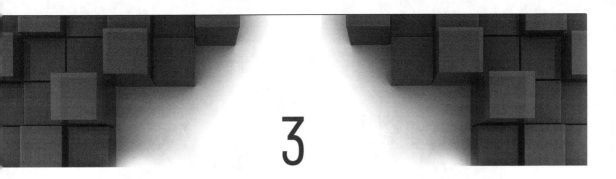

3

Keeping Current and Organizing Information on Research

*T*o be a competitive scientist, an investigator must remain constantly alert to new advances in the field as well as maintain access to previous research. At the outset, a doctoral student often is overwhelmed with new information. This makes it difficult to see the major issues and needs in a field. A doctoral dissertation usually is an offshoot of questions being addressed in the mentor's laboratory. The comprehensive examination often allows the candidate to select three to four areas that are related to his or her area of interest. The candidate is expected to become conversant with all of the major developments in each of these areas.

The first difficulty is information overload; everything seems to have equal importance. As the scientist becomes more knowledgeable in a field, the major trends become more evident. One way to start seeing these major issues or trends is to read recent review articles in the areas of interest to the student. Such reviews often point out the major issues that need to be addressed in the future and may indicate an area that the student wants to pursue. Attending doctoral seminars or journal clubs and scientific meetings often allows students to begin to identify the questions they plan to pursue in the future.

Access to new information is rarely a problem, organizing and managing it often is. This process is illustrated in Figure 3–1. You will need to have a bibliographic database(s) of references that you regularly use while reviewing research and writing manuscripts. This is paired with an electronic library of research articles that can be retrieved easily and read. From the bibliographic databases, you can search for relevant articles on a topic and then if the .pdf of an article is stored on your computer, you can easily read and refer to it as needed.

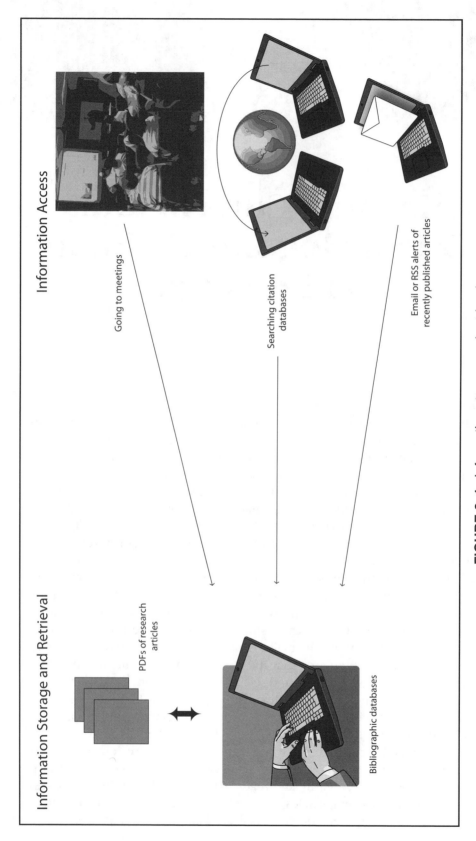

FIGURE 3–1. Information storage and retrieval.

Access to recent research is through online scientific data bases of published research in journals. Usually, articles can be downloaded from links attached to references within these databases onto your computer. In addition, regular updates can be provided by either E-mail or RSS feeds (which stands for "RDF site summary" or "really simple syndication"). RSS feeds come to your desktop on particular topics so that recent articles published in your area of interest will not be missed. You will need to have an RSS feed reader to receive these. These usually include the article citation and abstracts of an issue as soon as it is published. Also, you usually can request online publication (e-pub) alerts of articles that are "in press," which usually occur several months before an article is published in a journal. Many journals will send you tables of contents (TOC) alerts to your E-mail.

Another important source of new information is scientific meetings where you learn about others doing research in your field and seminal articles often are referred to in presentations. You can retrieve those articles from online data bases and .pdfs from journals. Each of these components is referred to in greater detail in this chapter.

BIBLIOGRAPHIC DATABASES

First is the need for bibliographic software to organize citations for easy citation during manuscript writing and developing bibliographies. Software programs support the development of a database of references to research articles, books and chapters, monographs, government publications, and so forth. Examples are EndNote© (http://www.endnote.com), Reference Manager© (http://www.refman.com), and ProCite® (http://www.procite.com). All three are purchased from Thomson Reuters and are very similar. References can easily be downloaded into the database from PubMed, Web of Science, and Scopus (see the section below on online research databases). You can search a topic, identify references, insert references into your bibliographic database, retrieve a copy of the published article, which can be linked to the citation in your bibliographic database, and the citation of the reference inserted into a manuscript as you write. Most of these database software packages are compatible with Microsoft Word©. The two programs interact so that, when you insert a reference into the text, the program automatically builds the bibliography in the style of the journal to which you plan to submit your article. As manuscripts are written, the references are automatically assembled in the correct style for the target journal. However, if the writer decides on a different journal or the manuscript is rejected and needs to be reformatted for a different journal, the citations immediately can be reassembled for another journal with different style requirements.

Having an up-to-date copy of bibliographic software is essential to making certain that your program has the correct style for each journal, so you should maintain updates for new versions. Establishing one large database with all of your references is best rather than small specific databases for each article. Most packages can easily handle at least 10,000 references. As you add references, change the date in the name of the database so that you are using a current version for a manuscript. Multiple copies are advisable as databases can become corrupted.

As manuscripts usually involve multiple authors who may draft various sections, sharing databases for constructing the bibliography is important. Two approaches can be used, either constructing a database unique to that article or sharing one database between all the authors. Alternatively, if everyone has access to a shared server, each person can add citations to the database and then download to create the links between the section he or she is writing and the database. That way, when the final bibliography is run, all the citations are present and correctly linked. This becomes important particularly if the first submission is rejected and the bibliography has to be rerun in a different journal style for submission to a new journal.

MAINTAINING AN ELECTRONIC LIBRARY OF ARTICLES

Most articles are now available in .pdf format which requires Adobe® Reader® which can be downloaded free of charge (http://www.adobe.com/products/reader/). The best way to organize articles for easy retrieval on your computer is to have a folder with all .pdf files with articles named in one convention (i.e., by first author, key words or title, journal, and year). For example an article might be titled, "Robey Single subj designs aphasia research Neuropsy Rev 2008." Articles then can be organized easily and searched by author, keywords, journals, and years. You can manually link .pdfs to citations in your bibliographic database. However, most bibliographic software packages download citation links into a bibliographic database from the online searches of data bases such as PubMed. While you are in your bibliographic software, for example, a search in PubMed will retrieve citations and automatically import them into your database. Other software such as QUOSA also can automatically retrieve article .pdfs during a search from databases such as PubMed, reducing a step. As long as your institution subscribes to journals electronically, you will be able to access the .pdf easily; otherwise, you will be charged for downloading the article, which may cost around 10 dollars.

ATTENDING SCIENTIFIC MEETINGS

Keeping track of research before or as it is published on the topics you are researching in your laboratory is essential. Going to meetings is important for staying ahead of what is going on before publication. Usually, there is at least a 1- to 2-year lag between the presentation of a new finding at a meeting and publication in a journal. Often attending one meeting per year is supported for doctoral and certainly for postdoctoral fellows. Going to scientific meetings is the best way to learn who else is working in the same area and might have recently completed studies that are being performed in your laboratory. An investigator should not spend time doing something that was already completed by someone else. Reading abstracts from meetings that have been held but could not be attended also is important.

AUTOMATED LITERATURE RETRIEVAL

Literature searches are essential to keeping up to date as a scientist. PubMed is the free online bibliographic service provided by the National Library of Medicine (NLM) and can be easily searched using terms that will be in the title or abstract and is free of charge (http://www.ncbi.nlm.nih.gov/sites/entrez?db =pubmed) (Figure 3–2). It includes biomedical research published in English as well as abstracts in English of articles published internationally in other languages. The NLM reviews journals and accepts only peer-reviewed biomedical research journals that are published regularly, such as on a quarterly basis. Consideration also is given to the size of the readership and relevance to biomedical researchers in selecting journals for PubMed. The publisher must apply to the NLM for inclusion; this can be time consuming and needs to address specific issues. Generally, PubMed requires not only that journals are peer reviewed and published reliably, but also that the content is of interest to scientists in

---

Boolean Searching

A single term retrieves all citations with the word either in the title, key words or abstract, e.g., stroke = 141,506 retrieved citations

Use of "and" restricts the search to only items that include both words, e.g., stroke + recovery = 8,018 citations

Use of "or" includes items that has either term,
e.g., stroke or recovery = _____ citations

Authors "Smith, A." will include all persons with that name and initial regardless of what other initials they have , e.g., Smith A = 10,905 while Smith AR = 370 citations

Combining terms "(stroke + recovery) + (rehabilitation)" = 2,371 citations.

FIGURE 3–2. Methods for constructing literature searches.

biomedical research, physicians, and other health care professionals. Some articles from journals thought to be from the social sciences, statistics, or engineering may not be included. However, PubMed is often slower to list article citations than some commercial databases such as Web of Science and Scopus.

Because most journals now do "e-pub" ahead of publication, searches will alert you to articles coming out many months before publication. "E-pub" usually becomes available shortly after an article is accepted, and if your institution subscribes to that journal, you will be able to download the accepted manuscript in advance of publication many months before the published .pdf is available.

Web of Science is provided as a retrieval service by the Institute of Scientific Information (ISI) Web of Knowledge published by Thomson Reuters. The ISI Web of Knowledge contains citations from the biological, medical, and social sciences and is available only if subscribed to by an institution or an individual, which can be costly. It contains citations to psychology and the social sciences to a greater degree than PubMed, which is more biomedical in focus. One limitation of Web of Science is the restricted searching capability by author by key word by year, reducing the ability to design searches that are more complex. Two other features of information, which are not available from PubMed, are available from Web of Science: the citations index and journal impact scores (based on the numbers of citations of articles in a journal). The numbers of citations is useful for identifying articles of high relevance to others doing research in that they have been cited in others' bibliographies. Similar to PubMed, citations can be saved directly to bibliographic data bases such as EndNote, Reference Manager, and Pro Cite data from retrieved records. Web of Science also does weekly retrieval alerts (see below) that are sent to a subscriber's E-mail address that include the abstract and links to the full citation if subscribed to by the institution.

Scopus is another commercially available retrieval service published by Elsevier that is often subscribed to by institutions. It includes over 16,000 peer-reviewed journals from more than 4,000 publishers, conference proceedings, trade publications, and book series. It also includes open access journals (see below) and both the biomedical and social sciences literature. Articles often are cited earlier in Scopus than in other databases. This retrieval service also provides numbers of citations of articles and can provide RSS feeds for regular retrievals in areas of interest to be sent to your desktop. Searching for an author only allows one initial, which limits the ability to confine the search to one author and is a limitation relative to PubMed (see Figure 3-2).

AUTOMATIC RETRIEVAL OF LITERATURE ON TOPICS

Weekly searches can also be conducted and delivered to your E-mail address of articles published in the journals cited by PubMed, which includes most national and international journals. The same is available from Web of Science and Scopus if your institution subscribes to those services. University or institutional libraries often provide links to the electronic version of the journal and the .pdf for the article on the citation if they subscribe to the electronic version of the journal. However, a recent move has been to make biomedical research accessible online free of charge, particularly when the research was supported by the United States Government or by charitable trusts such as the Welcome Trust in Britain. This is referred to as free access and is a rapidly increasing trend causing a revolution in publishing.

FREE ACCESS

Any research that was supported by grant funding from the National Institutes of Health (NIH) in the United States must be available online free of charge in PubMed Central (http://www.pubmedcentral.nih.gov/). Some journals have negotiated a 12-month delay in free access, referred to as the embargo period, but all research supported by NIH funds must be made available through PubMed Central (PMC) within 12 months of being published in a journal. This policy started in May 2004 and at first was voluntary; in 2008, it became mandatory that all NIH-supported investigators must register their articles in PubMed Central within 12 months of publication.

The Wellcome Trust (http://www.wellcome.ac.uk/), a charity in the United Kingdom that funds biomedical research in Britain and internationally, has a similar policy; all research supported by the Wellcome Trust must be available free of charge online to anyone after acceptance for publication (http://www .wellcome.ac.uk/About-us/Policy/Spotlight-issues/Open-access/Policy/ index.htm). The UK PubMed Central is a collaboration between the Wellcome Trust and the NIH (http://ukpmc.ac.uk/).

OPEN ACCESS JOURNALS

A recent innovation has been the development of online open access journals. These journals are published only online. In fact, fewer and fewer journals are published in hard copy, which reduces costs considerably. Open access journals provide accepted articles fre ely accessible online. A listing of these journals is available at (http://www.doaj.org/). For that reason, the cost of publication is borne by the authors and less by the publisher because there is no charge for access to the publication. The Public Library of Science (PLoS) is a nonprofit organization of scientists and physicians committed to making the world's scientific and medical literature a freely available public resource (http://www.plos.org/journals/index.php). PLoS journals are becoming popular; however, authors usually pay a substantial amount of the cost in the form of article processing fees while making access to the publications free of charge (Doyle, Gass, & Kennison, 2004a, 2004b). Other open access publishers are BioMed Central (BMC) journals (http://www.biomed-central.com/info/about/), which charge article processing fees somewhere between $1000 and $2000 per article. Bentham Science Publishers, Ltd., is another open access publisher who advertises lower cost article processing fees but also charges memberships at an average of $2000 per year with a 10% discount in the article publishing fee, making this a very costly alternative.

The HighWire Press® site available through Stanford University provides access to government publications and publications from journals participating that allow free online access for articles that are past the embargo period (http://highwire.stanford.edu/lists/largest.dtl). This is a new site listing all the HighWire Press journals that have agreed to participate. Oxford Open is a similar site for Oxford Press journals listing which journals have PubMed Central articles available free of charge but it is much less developed.

All of these changes in open access publishing for biomedical research have occurred rapidly over the last three years and are continuing to develop. Recently, some concerns have been expressed about the quality of the peer-review system for some of the open access journals. Rumors of fake articles being published have been damaging but need to be substantiated. Errors are to be expected with any new system and some changes should be expected over the next few years as these new journals mature.

If there is to be open access, how the cost of publishing research will be borne, is not clear. Traditional publishers still charge subscription fees from university and research institution libraries; however, these have become very costly, taking a larger and larger share of the support costs for research out of university budgets. This has led to the move for open access publishing particularly as the support for biomedical research in many countries is from taxpayer dollars, and some express the concern that taxpayers who support biomedical research should have free and open access to the results of that research. As a result, publishers are now moving toward charging authors "article processing fees," which are high and cannot be paid except from grants reducing the monies available to support research. This has led to the concern that new scientists, particularly those without research grant support, will not have the funds to pay the costs for article processing fees. As such they will be the disenfranchised from the science world, making it particularly difficult for new investigators to publish at a time in their career when publication is critical to future success (Doyle et al., 2004b). At this point, it is not clear what solutions will be found to this dilemma and how open access will be maintained.

Surveys of scientists' opinions regarding open access have shown that many are not aware of the transition that is rapidly taking place and that many are unaware of the pending change in asking scientists to support the cost of publication (Schroter, 2006; Schroter & Tite, 2006). Over the next couple of years, some solutions that could provide relief for the new investigators particularly at small institutions probably will emerge.

KEEPING UP WITH FUNDED RESEARCH

The National Institutes of Health provides RePORTER (http://projectreporter .nih.gov/reporter.cfm), an online database that allows retrieval of all grants funded including both research and research training grants. This is an improved search system replacing CRISP, which provides additional information on funded research. It can be searched by funding institute, principal investigator, key words, and grant type. When writing grant applications it is always advisable to search funded research in your area of interest before progressing too far on an application. It is best to distinguish your grant from those that are funded so your proposal will appear unique, an important issue to NIH program staff. Interesting aspects are the ability to retrieve information on the funds being spent in selected areas of research such as disease categories.

The increased emphasis in the NIH grant system for determining the innovation and significance of the research being proposed places an increased burden on investigators proposing their research. They must have a comprehensive grasp of the current literature and funded research to demonstrate that their research addresses not only an important problem but is unique, ground breaking, and of significance to the health of Americans. Sifting through the increasing volume of research literature to make this case is no small endeavor.

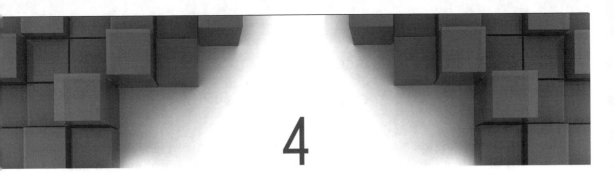

4

Writing and Publishing Scientific Papers

WHAT IS A SCIENTIFIC RESEARCH PAPER?

This is such a basic question that the answer seems obvious, but it is helpful to define this term carefully as a foundation for this chapter. According to the Council of Biology Editors (which became the Council of Science Editors on January 1, 2000), a scientific research paper is defined by three criteria (Council of Biology Editors, 1968; as cited by Day, 1994, p. 9).

1. It is the first publication of a scientific result.

2. It constitutes a report that contains sufficient information so that peers can assess observations, repeat experiments and evaluate intellectual processes.

3. It appears in a journal or other resource readily available to the scientific community (and often the public at large).

These three criteria not only define a scientific paper as a product of science but they also denote critical aspects of science in a more general sense, namely, the aspects of discovery, evaluation and replication, and dissemination.

This chapter describes how scientific papers are prepared, submitted for publication in a refereed journal, and reviewed in the journal's editorial process. Issues of publication ethics, which are fundamental to the integrity of science, are interwoven with general information on scientific publishing, on the assumption that every decision should be made with due regard to ethical standards.

GENERAL GUIDELINES

The general approach to scientific writing outlined here is indexed to the IMRAD format (Sollaci & Pereira, 2004). IMRAD is an acronym for *i*ntroduction, *m*ethod, *r*esults, *a*nd *d*iscussion, which is the standard used in scientific writing. This structure is endorsed by scientific organizations and by nearly all biomedical journals. The scientist who prepares a paper with an eye toward IMRAD is following a tradition in scientific writing that reaches back to the 17th century. Before that time, scientific reports typically took a form of a letter in which a scientist shared results of experiments.

One reason sometimes given for the IMRAD structure is that if follows the basic sequence of steps in a scientific investigation. However, science does not always proceed in such a steplike fashion, and a more important reason for this format is that the modular organization permits readers to scan quickly for the information that is most important to them. IMRAD lends a degree of predictability to scientific papers, so that the reader can peruse a paper with high efficiency. (A good source on IMRAD is: The basics of writing a paper, available from http://bmj.bmjjournals.com/talks/wjournal/).

Although the following discussion basically follows the sequence of sections in a published paper, it should be emphasized that this sequence is rarely followed when writing a paper. For example, most authors write the abstract only after the bulk of the paper is complete to be sure that the abstract reflects the work as a whole. Similarly, the title often is decided only after the paper is essentially complete. There is no hard and fast rule on the order of steps in writing a paper. This is a matter of both individual preference and the nature of the research. A common recommendation is to write the methods section first, because it is pivotal to the research at hand. Often organizing the results section before writing the introduction and discussion can be helpful.

Title and Introduction

The introduction consists of the title, author listing, abstract, and the introduction proper. The title may be the most important phrase in the article. Generally, the title should be fully explanatory when it stands alone. But it should be economical, expressing its content in as few words as possible. Overly long, jargon-laden titles can be impenetrable to some potential readers and offensive to others. Simplicity and economy go together to define an effective title. The title fulfills two main information functions: (a) it informs readers about the article, and (b) it is used in indexing the article in the journal's index as well as in abstracting and literature search systems. For some journals, an abbreviated title known as the running title appears on each published page. The title serves other functions as well. In a curriculum vitae (CV) (see Chapter 10), an individual's publications are listed by author, title, and journal information. Therefore, the CV is a profile of scientific productivity, and titles of papers help to summarize important aspects of a research career.

Authorship

Who should be listed as an author of a scientific paper? Attempts to answer this question penetrate into the nature of individual responsibility for scientific effort and discovery. There is no simple answer, but there are responsible ways of coming to an answer that provide general guidance and assurance to all concerned. The word "author" is derived from the Latin word *auctor*, meaning "creator, originator." The word "authority" comes from the same root, and it is no accident that an author of scientific or scholarly publications often is recognized as an authority or expert on the subject. In more modern thinking, the term "intellectual property" is an issue related to creativity or originality, and the importance of this concept is one reason for the growth of intellectual property as a legal specialty.

According to the International Committee of Medical Journal Editors (ICMJE; http://www.icmje.org/) criteria (Garcia, 2004), three conditions must be met for any individual to be listed as an author of a scientific paper. First, the individual must have made substantial contributions to conception and design, or acquisition of data, or analysis and interpretation of data. Second, the individual should have played a major role in drafting the article or revising it critically for important intellectual content. And, third, the individual should have expressed final approval of the version to be published (Figure 4–1).

Requirements for Authorship
International Council of Journal Medical Editors

- Substantial contributions to:
  - conception and design, or
  - acquisition of data, or
  - analysis and interpretation of data
- Play a major role in drafting the articles or revising it critically for important intellectual content
- Expressed final approval of the version to be published

FIGURE 4–1. Requirements for authorship based on the International Council of Journal Medical Editors.

These basic criteria are valuable standards in deciding on authorship and they are the principles for the continuing discussion of this topic.

The main author of a paper, usually the first or senior author and designated as the corresponding author, bears special responsibility. No matter the number of authors on a paper, one individual should be accountable for the decision/decisions and actions that underlie the published article. The main author should pay careful attention to all aspects of the process and should be in a position to answer any questions that may arise. It is not taking the responsibility too far for the first author to answer satisfactorily the three questions posed in the preceding paragraph for each author of a paper.

A variety of individuals sit on the margins of authorship as defined above: "ghostwriter" authors, honorary authors, gift authors, and coercion authors. Ghostwriters write much or all of the text in an article, and often are paid for their verbal skills. However, they typically have little or nothing to do with the scientific process itself and rarely are involved until the final paper is prepared. They may lack the expertise to explain or defend decision regarding research design and data interpretation. Large research projects may hire ghostwriters to give final polish to journal articles, research grant applications, and other documents. Ethical principles for professional writers are discussed by Jacobs et al. (2005). Honorary authors may be laboratory directors, supervisors, mentors, or colleagues who have not participated significantly in the research—not satisfying the ICMJE criteria outlined above—but are granted author status nonetheless as a token of respect to their position or overall support. It is sometimes said, not necessarily facetiously, that the two prominent positions of authorship are the first and the last in an author list. According to this assertion, the first author is credited with the major inspiration and effort, whereas the last author is the head of the laboratory. Gift authors are just that—they receive authorship as a gift for reasons that may be known only to the other authors, or even only the main author. Coercion authors are those who have authorship forced on them, even if they have no real involvement with the underlying science and do not necessarily desire authorship. Valuable discussions of general authorship considerations are available (Benos et al., 2005; Claxton, 2005).

Much is at stake in scientific authorship (Claxton, 2005). Publications establish a record of productivity, justify funding for research, create reputations of individual scientists and research teams, and build careers. Science is influential mainly through publications that advance knowledge, and individual scientists are known largely for their publications in refereed journals.

Particularly in scientific and technical fields, the number of authors on publications has been increasing as the complexity of research questions has grown, as multidisciplinary research has flourished, and as research teams or collaborations expand. "Authorship issues are increasing, primarily because the average number of authors per research article has been steadily rising over the years" (Benos et al., 2005). Multiple authorship of a paper also creates a potential ethical problem (Lazer, 2004). It is common now to see seven or more authors on a scientific publication. One risk of multiple authorships is that responsibility is diffused to the point of no responsibility at all, although each author has the same responsibility for ensuring the scientific integrity of the research.

Not everyone who contributes to a scientific publication deserves to be an author. Some should be mentioned in an acknowledgment for their assistance. Authorship versus acknowledgment can be a weighty decision. It can be difficult to avoid "intellectual exploitation" (Martin, 1992) while keeping true to the standard of credible authorship. In many research projects, a considerable effort is made by lab assistants, librarians, biostatisticians, and others who may be neglected from mention of any kind. An argument often made against including these individuals in the authorship of a paper is that they do their circumscribed duties under the supervision of one or more scientists who bear the ultimate responsibility for the research project. Someone who searches the literature on a topic, collects data in a predetermined protocol, or does limited data analysis with prescribed methods does not satisfy the three criteria for authorship stated earlier in this chapter. Authorship should not extend to every individual who contributes to a scientific project, and it is an ethical responsibility of the main author to be able to defend the inclusion of all authors on an article and to explain the role of those who are acknowledged for their assistance.

Final decisions on some aspects of authorship of a paper may have to wait until the paper is ready to submit for publication. Sometimes a preliminary plan for a paper is altered drastically as the paper comes to reality, and the changes may increase or decrease the contribution of any one individual. For example, suppose that a biostatistician originally was expected to play a central role because of a novel statistical analysis that was crucial to the project. However, the planned analysis was dropped in favor of a more conventional approach that could be implemented with readily available software and little advice from the biostatistician. In such a circumstance, the biostatistician might be dropped from authorship of the paper. Consider another scenario: a colleague with substantial expertise on the topic of a paper is asked to review a draft of the paper before it is submitted for publication. This colleague makes sweeping suggestions for revision, including a recommendation for a complete reanalysis of the data that permits a critical test of a prevailing theory. In recognition of such a profound contribution, the colleague may be invited to be a coauthor. This being said, it usually is a good idea to determine as early as possible who the authors will be and in what order their names will appear. Ill feelings can develop if one of the scientists contributing to a project has expectations that are not shared by the other authors. It is difficult to lay down hard and fast rules for the order of authors. Ideally, a discussion among all those concerned will be sufficient to determine the order. But, if disagreements arise, it is wise to try to settle the issue well before the paper is drafted, allowing that reconsideration may be needed as the work progresses. When contributions to a paper are essentially equal, the authors may agree to an alphabetical listing or simply drawing straws to determine order of authorship. Some published papers mention specifically how the order of authorship was determined, especially in cases of nearly equal contributions to the science.

Abstract

The title of an article might catch a reader's attention but a well-crafted abstract can turn that attention into genuine interest for further reading. Van Way (2007) asserted that, "Abstract preparation is a minor art form in itself" (p. 638). For research articles, the abstract should describe the problem, subject, method, major result(s), and conclusions. Abstracts fall into two basic types: structured and unstructured. Structured abstracts are prepared with distinct, labeled sections. They summarize a scientific paper by using fixed categories such as objective, methods, results, and conclusions. Such uniformity in design of the abstract aids the reader in gathering the main information about a paper and is especially helpful for indexing and literature retrieval purposes. The headings of a structured abstract vary somewhat across journals. For example, alternatives to the example given above are: (a) context, background, aim, findings, interpretation and (b) design, population, setting, participants, intervention (method), and main outcome measures. Journals usually specify the kind of abstract that is required.

Unstructured abstracts allow the author(s) to determine what kind of summary is appropriate. The freedom given to authors carries the risk that abstracts will vary according to individual bias and choice. An author who prepares an unstructured abstract usually is not given guidance on the substance of the abstract and may emphasize any aspect of the article, even to the exclusion of information that is critical in structured abstracts. One problem with these abstracts is that they sometimes lead the reader to a misleading impression of the significance of the paper.

Structured abstracts originally were used in clinical research, but they are now favored by many journals in a variety of disciplines and fields and are increasingly used in scientific and technical journals. See Kostoff and Hartley (2001) for a discussion of the advantages of these abstracts for purposes such as data mining. Journals also may require the author to submit a small number of keywords to be used in indexing (Kostoff & Hartley, 2001). These should be identified thoughtfully because they can direct the literature retrieval process. They should not include terms already in the title or abstract as these are also used for searching in most online scientific databases.

The Body of the Paper

The introduction, methods, results, and discussion comprise the body of the paper. These sections should be cohesive and logical in their development. An hourglass analogy is useful in getting a perspective on how the body should be written. The top of the hourglass is a wide funnel, corresponding to the introduction that gives a general context for the research to be reported. The narrow waist of the hour glass corresponds to the methods and results that are highly specific to the particular research being reported. The hour glass expands in its lower section, analogous to the discussion that evaluates and interprets the research in the larger context of investigation and theory. The paper usually has a circular structure insofar as the discussion examines and resolves issues raised in the introduction. Now we take a closer look at each section of the body.

The Introduction Proper

The statement of the problem is a concise formulation of the central issue addressed in the paper. This statement gives perspective on the research at hand, and ideally it unifies the specific purposes to lay a foundation for the conclusions and interpretation.

The rationale for the study: (1) gives the reasons for the research, (2) justifies the selection of independent and dependent variables, population(s) under study, and (3) may explain the methods of research. It is never sufficient as a rationale to say that the study has not been done. Hundreds of studies have not been done. A satisfactory rationale establishes the need for the study on legitimate scientific grounds. A compelling introduction commands the reader's attention.

The review of the literature develops the rationale for the study and places the research done in a scientific context. This portion of the paper can be a highly valuable part of the article that establishes the standard of scholarship and defines the state of the relevant science. Because most journals impose limits on the length of published articles, care should be taken to cite the most relevant literature and crystallize the important results of previous research. Selectivity runs counter to comprehensiveness, and emphasizing one necessarily sacrifices the other. This can be a difficult balance, which is one of the challenges in writing an effective introduction. Some journals favor (or even require) a very brief introduction that includes a minimum of references to the literature. The goal is to state as briefly as possible the purpose of the research. Review of the literature is saved for the discussion section.

The specific purposes, research questions, or hypotheses usually appear at the end of the introduction and they lead directly into the remainder of the article. The wording of these elements is highly important and should be tied very closely to the major results of the study.

Methods

It usually is best to begin with a description of the experimental design or study design. This information orients the reader to the major approach. Some or all of the following suggestions then may apply, depending on the type of research.

Research Participants: Animals or Human Subjects. The types of information that are usually critical to an assessment of the suitability of participants include: sample size (number of participants), inclusionary/exclusionary criteria used in selecting participants, attrition of participants (if applicable), and participant information (e.g., age, sex, disease, time since diagnosis). Inclusionary and exclusionary criteria should be clearly described. Description of participants can appear in either the methods or results section. Particularly for clinical research, some authors prefer to include participant information in the results section because the recruitment of subjects is a result of planned procedures and shapes the other results to be reported.

Materials. This category includes information on chemicals, special preparations, software, and hardware instrumentation (apparatus). For complicated or novel instrumentation, a block diagram should be used to describe the major components and their connections. If calibration was used, then information should be given on the purpose of calibration, equipment and procedures used, and when the calibration was done. It is appropriate to identify the manufacturer or vendor of commercially available materials.

Research Controls. This category depends on the kind of research. Generally speaking, any environmental variable that conceivably could affect the results of a study should be described along with efforts taken to control or minimize its influence.

Instructions to Participants or Training Research Participants. Specific to human research, directions to participants should be clearly stated. Frequently, if the instructions are brief, they can be included verbatim in the report. Otherwise, they can be placed in an appendix or added to the online journal as supplementary materials, on a Web site, or other readily available location.

Procedures. The steps taken in the experiment or study must be described to satisfy the criterion of replicability, that is, the assurance that another scientist with suitable competence in the discipline or laboratory techniques could repeat the research. In the case of complex research involving a number of steps, each step should be described. The experimental design should be specified, perhaps with justification for the selection of a particular design.

Animal Care and Use or Protection of Human Subjects. For research involving animals, the methods section typically ends with a statement of compliance with guidelines for animal experimentation and approval by the local Institutional Animal Care and Use Committee (IACUC). For research on humans, a statement is included to indicate approval by the Institutional Review Board (IRB). Some journals require that such statements be present before a paper can be accepted for publication. It is good practice to include this information in all research papers.

Results

No single template is used for writing the results section of a scientific paper, although some principles are fairly common across disciplines and topics. Careful thought should be given to the organization of the results so that the data are presented in the most efficient and understandable way. Statistical tables, summary tables, or graphs often are pivotal in this section because they summarize the data for deriving conclusions and interpretations. It often is recommended that the tables and figures or graphs be developed first and that the text be written with these in mind. Whatever the sequence, the text should be developed to give tables and graphs the importance they deserve. The reader should easily understand how the tables and figures or graphs relate to the text. A basic rule is that every table and figure should be mentioned in the text, ideally at a point in the text that invites the reader's attention to full advantage. Both tables and figures are numbered in succession based on where they were placed in the text.

Ideally, tables and figures should be as fully self-explanatory as possible. In the case of very complex tables or figures, it may be necessary to refer to the text for a full explanation. In general, it is not advisable to present the same information in tables and illustrations. In preparing illustrations, it is best to avoid "chartjunk" (vibrations, grids, and ducks) (Aydingoz, 2005; Schriger & Cooper, 2001; Tufte, 1983). Software programs allow users to generate a variety of embellishments. These encumber figures with graphic complexity obscuring the important information and are better left out. The goal is to present the results in an economical and effective way, so that every line and every symbol is judiciously chosen to portray the data.

Special care should be taken in the preparation of images to be reproduced in publication. Digital images are a boon to scientific publication and can be used for photomicrographs, blots, gels, magnetic resonance or x-ray images, and so on. Journals often will specify the essential requirements for images. Digital enhancement of images carries other risks. It is very easy to enhance an image to make it clearer, to delete parts of the image, or otherwise improve it. Some editors of scientific journals understandably are concerned that enhancements can cross the threshold into data falsification (discussed later in this chapter). The real world of science is often a bit messier than we might like it; we should be very careful not to use digital methods to bring nature up to our personal standards or to meet our expectations of a good result. Rossner and Yamada (2004) provide guidance on this matter, giving examples of how inappropriate manipulation of a digital image can affect micrographs, blots, and gels. Only limited adjustments are acceptable and it is advisable to disclose any such alterations to the readership. Hames (2008) states two basic rules to be followed in preparing digital images. First, images should be prepared with the least possible processing and should be an accurate representation of the acquired data. Second, digital effects that are used should be applied to the entire image and should never result in loss or selective enhancement of features (Hames, 2008). It always is a good idea to preserve a file of the original analog or digital data in case questions arise.

IMRAD describes the basic structure of a scientific paper that has served as the template for hundreds of thousands of articles. Depending on the kind of paper that is being prepared, other reporting guidelines may be followed. For particular kinds of papers in certain journals, these guidelines are necessary and must be followed as closely as possible. Some examples of guidelines are:

1. CONsolidated Standards Of Reporting Trials (CONSORT)—developed to guide standardized reporting of randomized clinical trials for pharmacologic research (Moher, Schulz, & Altman, 2001). An extension of the original CONSORT statement for trials assessing nonpharmacologic treatments was described (Boutron, Moher, Altman, Schulz, & Ravaud, 2008).

2. Transparent Reporting of Evaluations with Nonrandomized Designs (TREND)—developed to guide standardized reporting of nonrandomized controlled trials (Des Jarlais, Lyles, & Crepaz, 2004).

3. Standards for Reporting of Diagnostic Accuracy (STARD)—developed to guide the reporting of studies of diagnostic accuracy (Bossuyt et al., 2003).

4. Meta-analysis of observational studies in epidemiology (Stroup et al., 2000).

5. The quality of reporting meta-analyses of randomized controlled trials (Quality of Reporting of Meta-analyses, QUOROM) has been specified (Moher et al., 1999).

Discussion and Conclusions

The discussion considers the results of the study in light of the larger historical, theoretical, and empirical context. As such, this section of a paper is the intersection of discovery and interpretation. Many authors start with a concise statement of the major conclusions, ideally related to previous parts of the article to ensure effective closure and continuity. The results then are considered in relation to previous research to indicate points of agreement or disagreement, resolution or lack of it. Novel aspects of the current research can be emphasized, along with theoretical and practical implications. Although it is not always necessary to acknowledge limitations of the study being reported, comments along this line are helpful as cautionary notes to the reader and as a stimulus to future research. This section on limitations often can be used to address shortcomings that reviewers may identify. Similarly, it is not always necessary to specify implications for future research, but suggestions of this kind can be provocative.

References and Appendices

Generally, references to original research are preferred over references to review articles or secondary sources (Garcia, 2004). One reason is to give credit to those who first reported a scientific result. But a countervailing force is that some journals restrict the number of references in a given scientific article. Authors may find it convenient to cite a single review paper rather than original publications. Finding a compromise is not always easy. There are times when citing a review article is both economical and justified, such as when the article provides an illuminating synthesis of a subject. But if a review article provides little more than a list of papers germane to a topic, then it is more difficult to justify citation of the review article over citation of the original papers.

Authors are responsible for checking the accuracy of citations and interpretations of published articles. Generally, the reference list should be pruned to include only essential references, unless the purpose of the article dictates otherwise (e.g., the article is intended as a comprehensive review of a topic). Many journals place a limit on the number of references, so that the author(s) must decide which references are most important for the work at hand. Restricting the number of references can be difficult because it forces a trade-off between completeness of scholarship and the need for economical use of journal pages.

Papers should include references that have been carefully read, not simply because they can be easily inserted into a list to make the author look well-informed and diligent. Scientists should heed Chargaff's (1976) admonition against taking chunks of bibliographies "wafted in their entirety from one paper to the next"(Chargaff, 1976). Martin (1992) refers to cited publications as one of the common areas of scientific misrepresentation because the author of a paper may not have read the cited literature but nonetheless includes the references in conclusions or interpretations (Martin, 1992). Scientists are responsible not only for their own data but also for the use they make of previously published reports. One is reminded of one of Murphy's laws: the work that is cited inaccurately will have been written by one of the reviewers assigned to the paper at hand. Be forewarned!

OTHER KINDS OF ARTICLES AND PUBLICATIONS

There are few reliable guidelines for other kinds of articles, which usually do not follow the IMRaD format. Publishers' style manual may offer some advice. These articles include case reports (Chelvarajah & Bycroft, 2004; McCarthy & Reilly, 2000; Wright & Kouroukis, 2000); tutorials, critical reviews (Siwek, Gourlay, Slawson, & Shaughnessy, 2002); abstracts and posters (Boullata & Mancuso, 2007), and book or product reviews.

ADVICE ON WRITING

Scientific writing draws on a number of skills and abilities. Doing it well takes practice and commitment. Taking advice from experienced writers is a good way to polish writing. Some resources that may be helpful are: Brumback (2009); Editors (October 2008); Goldbort (1998); Kliewer (2005); Lang (2001) and Toft and Jaeger (1998); Van Way (2007); Webb (2002); White (2002). Probably the best advice on this matter is never to assume that the draft that satisfies your own standards is the best possible communication of your scientific effort. The sentence that you may think is brilliant and crystal clear may lead another reader to wonder what you are trying to say.

ETHICAL MATTERS

Plagiarism, Fabrication, and Falsification

"Becoming immensely rich is not a frequent risk among public health researchers" (Garcia, 2004). As true as this statement may be, it does not mean that scientists are immune to temptations and ethical dilemmas as they conduct and report their research. Ethical breaches occur across economic strata. Temptations surrounding reputation, grant funding, promotion, patents, and other markers of success may lead scientists into unethical behavior. Although such behavior may be rare, science should expect zero tolerance when it comes to ethical breaches. Scientific misconduct according to the U.S. Dept. of Health and Human Services (1990) takes three major forms: *Plagiarism* involves presenting another's ideas without attribution. *Fabrication* is presenting unsubstantiated facts for data. *Falsification* is altering or selecting certain data to achieve a desired result, misrepresenting evidence, facts, or authorship.

Other Serious Deviations from Accepted Practice in Proposing, Conducting or Reporting Research

Redundant Publication

Redundant or repetitive publication is defined as "the publication of copyrighted material with additional new or unpublished data" (Benos, et al., 2005, p. 63). There are many reasons why redundant publication is damaging to science:

1. It may infringe international copyright law.

2. It is a poor use of reviewers' time and precious journal pages.

3. It adds to a literature that is often large already and difficult to review.

4. It fragments rather than unifies data from a closely related group.

5. It may give undeserved weight to a study by reporting the results more than once.

6. It can compromise the value of subsequent meta-analysis by inflating patient or experimental numbers.

Duplicate Publication

Duplicate publication, or self-plagiarism, is defined as "the publication of an article that is identical or overlaps substantially with an article already published elsewhere, with or without acknowledgment" (Benos et al., 2005, p. 63). A primary reason why duplicate publication is objectionable is that it has the potential to "skew the evidence base" (Benos et al., 2005). Journals discourage the practice of duplicate publication by prohibiting the simultaneous submission of a manuscript to more than one journal. APA specifically forbids concurrent submission of manuscripts.

Conflict of Interest

This is a complex topic that is considered elsewhere in this book. The primary relevance of the topic to scientific publications is disclosure and transparency. The Council of Science Editors (CSE) defines on its Web site (http://www.councilscienceeditors.org/services/draft_approved.cfm) conflict of interest in regard to scientific publishing as "sets of conditions in which an author, editor, or reviewer holds conflicting or competing interests that could result in bias or improper decisions. The conflicts of interest may only be potential conflicts of interest or only perceived, and not necessarily even potential, conflicts." This definition places a considerable burden on all involved to be sensitive to conflicts of interest, even perceived conflicts of interest, and to guard against any bias or influence of these circumstances on the work in question. In a systematic review of studies on financial conflict of interest in research, it was concluded that there was: (a) a statistically significant relationship between industry sponsorship and pro-industry conclusions, and (b) an association between industry sponsorship and restrictions on publication and data sharing (Bekelman, Li, & Gross, 2003).

The key points to remember are: objectivity is the standard to be achieved; financial and other interests should be disclosed; and transparency of connections among authors, reviewers, publishers, editors, and funding sources must be maintained (L. Friedman & Richter, 2005).

Financial interests include some that are obvious, such as stock ownership, board membership, paid employment, and gifts. Others that are sometimes overlooked are patent applications, research grants, travel or conference grants, and honoraria for talks or attendance at meetings. Personal interests include membership in lobbying organizations, or personal relationships with editors or with individuals who may be asked to review the paper. Professional interests include service on a federal advisory board, service as an expert witness, writing for an educational or publishing company, or having a relationship with funding agencies.

Animal Welfare Concerns; Human Use Concerns

Universities and research institutions require that investigators complete training in the ethics of research involving animals and human participants. Research protocols are evaluated by an Institutional Review Board (IRB) or Institutional Animal Care and Use Committee (IACUC), and investigators/investigations can proceed with their research only when the protocol is approved. As noted earlier in the discussion of the methods section on preparing a paper, many scientific articles include a statement that the research protocol was approved by the IRB or IACUC. But whether such a statement is included in the published article or not, the principal investigator must maintain a file of communications from the appropriate review committees.

Who Bears Responsibility for Ethics?

There is a chain of responsibility for research ethics that includes the investigators who author and submit papers for publication, journal editors and manuscript reviewers, IRBs, and funding sources. All authors of an article must assume responsibility, particularly because they generally are the ones to initiate an ethical breach. It appears that ethical violations are not equal in the minds of scientists. Korenman et al. (1998) used a mailed survey consisting of 12 scenarios in 4 domains of research ethics to determine how scientists weighed the severity of ethical misconduct (Korenman, Berk, & Lew, 1998). Respondents were asked to determine if an act was unethical and, if so, to rate the degree to which they thought it was unethical, and to select responses and punishments for the act. The most serious offenses were fabrication, falsification, and plagiarism. Moderately serious offenses included misleading statements about a paper and failure to give proper attribution. The following were in a category of less serious offenses: sloppiness, oversight, conflict of interest, and failure to share.

Reviewers of manuscripts submitted for journal publication often are in a good position to detect breaches of research ethics. Atlas (2003) suggested that editors provide instructions to authors on the following: (a) overarching ethical guidelines, (b) protecting patient/subject rights, (c) protecting animal welfare, (d) conflicts of interest, (e) publication issues, and (f) professional cooperation (Atlas, 2003).

Funding sources also must be vigilant with regard to research ethics. At the minimum, they should ensure that research they support has received appropriate review and approval by an IRB. Progress reports should be reviewed with attention to standards of ethical research.

IRBs obviously have a major role, and are often a first line of protection, in guarding against unethical research procedures. Because IRB approval is required before a research project begins, questionable procedures often can be identified in time to advise the researcher of the problems and perhaps to recommend solutions.

What Are the Most Common Unethical Behaviors?

Martinson et al. (2005) conducted a survey of scientists to determine the frequency of occurrence for various kinds of unethical behavior (Martinson, Anderson, & de Vries, 2005). Their results indicated that the least frequent ethical breaches (those with less than 2% frequency of occurrence) were: falsifying or "cooking" research data; ignoring major aspects of human-subject requirements; not properly disclosing involvement in firms whose products are based on one's own research; relationships with students, research subjects, or clients that may be interpreted as questionable; using another's ideas without obtaining permission or giving due credit; and unauthorized use of confidential information in connection with one's own research. More frequent behaviors were: failing to present data that contradict one's own previous research (6.0%); circumventing certain minor aspects of human-subject requirements (7.6%); overlooking others' use of flawed data or questionable interpretation of data (12.5%) and changing the design, methodology, or results of a study in response to pressure from a funding source (15.5%). For a discussion of ethical issues related to biostatistics, see Ranstam et al. (2000).

What Is Done When Ethical Violations Are Reported or Suspected?

Helpful recommendations are found in COPE (1999) and Benos et al. (2005). Sanctions in rough order of severity are:

1. Letter of explanation to authors, where there appears to be a genuine misunderstanding of principles.

2. A letter of reprimand and warning as to future conduct.

3. A formal letter to the relevant head of institution or funding body.

4. Publication of a notice of redundant publication or plagiarism.

5. An editorial giving full details of the misconduct.

6. Refusal to accept future submissions from the individual, unit, or institution responsible for the misconduct, for a stated period.

7. Formal withdrawal or retraction of the paper from the scientific literature, informing other editors and the indexing authorities.

8. Reporting the case to the General Medical Council, or other such authority or organization that can investigate and act with due process.

Corrections and Retractions

Like all human endeavor, science is liable to errors, omissions, and failure to certify accuracy. Sadly, tracking these failings is a difficult task that often takes months or years and has uncertain consequences, as discussed by Eysenbach and Kummervold (2005) and P. J. Friedman (1990). The National Library of Medicine's practices for handling errata and retractions were described by Kotzin and Schuyler (1989). Retraction is defined as "a letter to the editor or an editorial stating that an article previously published was based on fraudulent research, that is, research in which deliberately falsified or unsubstantiated data were used" (Kotzin & Schuyler, 1989, p. 337). Errata are "significant errors in the text, abstract, or descriptive part of an article" (Kotzin & Schuyler, 1989, p. 339). According to Kotzin and Schuyler, indexers found as many as 200 substantive errata each month. With the increase in the number of published articles today relative to 1989, the number of errata must be staggering. A major problem is that both retractions and errata, when published, can be difficult to link to the original article, so that readers may not know that a published article is subject to these actions. Unfortunately, journals do not always have written procedures for responding to allegations of research misconduct (P. J. Friedman, 1990).

Unintentional Misrepresentation in Science

It is easy to be smug and self-content about scientific fraud. But as Medawar (1963) and Martin (1992) warn, the process of science is often perilously close to misrepresentation. Medawar remarked that, " . . . the scientific paper is a fraud in the sense that it does give a totally misleading narrative of the processes of thought that go into the making of scientific discoveries" (Medawar, 1990, p. 16). Martin goes so far as to say that misrepresentation is nearly impossible to avoid:

> [The scientific paper] presents a mythical reconstruction of what actually happened. All of what are in retrospect mistaken ideas, badly designed experiments and incorrect calculations are omitted. The paper presents the research as if it had been carefully thought out, planned and executed according to a neat, rigorous process, for example involving testing of a hypothesis. (Martin, 1992, p. 85)

Martin gives the example of the *striking* contrast between the famous Watson and Crick paper published in *Nature* in 1953, and Watson's book accounting the discovery of the structure of DNA, *The Double Helix* (Martin, 1992). *Spontaneous Apprentices* by the psychologist George Miller also gives the unpolished side of science—the challenges and adjustments that rarely are hinted at in published scientific articles (Miller, 1977). Scientific papers generally make research studies appear to be much cleaner and more straightforward than they actually are. Fortunately, the method of science is robust enough to overcome the discrepancy between the actual practice of science and the published product. Published scientific articles usually are done in a standardized way that facilitates the dissemination of information, and not to reflect the variations in how research is conducted. This assertion is made only to show that orthodoxy in publication does not need to have provenance in the research method per se. The process of discovery is not isomorphic with the process of dissemination, but both have legitimacy in their principles.

Negative Results

Much of the work of science is never seen in print. This is particularly so for the dreaded "negative result." The exclusion of such research from the literature raises a number of issues pertaining to replication and wasted effort ("If I had known someone had tried that and failed, it would have saved me both time and money"). Negative results are a natural and unavoidable part of science, which is perhaps why new journals are appearing that unabashedly publish the heretofore unpublishable. Witness the *Journal of Negative Results in BioMedicine* and the *Journal of Negative Results in Speech and Audio Sciences*. The former invites contributions as follows with this statement on its Web page (http://www.jnrbm.com/):

> Journal of Negative Results in BioMedicine is ready to receive papers on all aspects of unexpected, controversial, provocative and/or negative results/conclusions in the context of current tenets, providing scientists and physicians with responsible and balanced information to support informed experimental and clinical decisions.

As Smith (2006) points out, studies that find a treatment to be effective tend to be published more than once, whereas studies that find a treatment not to be effective, are not published at all (Smith, 2006). The result is a systematic bias that favors effective treatments out of proportion to their actual value. In recognition of this biasing effect, the Web page of the ICMJE (http://www .icmje.org/) has the following to say about publication of negative results:

> Editors should consider seriously for publication any carefully done study of an important question, relevant to their readers, whether the results for the primary or any additional outcome are statistically significant. Failure to submit or publish findings because of lack of statistical significance is an important cause of publication bias. (Editors, October 2008)

The recent requirement that all clinical trials (either funded by the NIH, foundations, or industry) are registered in http://clinicaltrials.gov/ and that the results are made available on that Web site 1 year following the completion of data collection will go a long way to address this problem (see Chapter 11).

Peer Review

Scientific peer review generally is defined as the evaluation of research findings for competence, significance, and originality by qualified experts. Peer review is intended to ensure that the scientific literature is accurate, dependable, and clear. Of course, peer review, like all facets of science, is a human endeavor and it suffers from occasional failings as well as successes (Benos et al., 2007; Vanrooyan, 1990). Nonetheless, it has served science well. Apparently the first peer-reviewed collection of medical articles appeared in 1731, with the publication of *Medical Essays and Observations* by the Royal Society of Edinburgh. But peer review of scientific papers really took hold after World War II as scientific productivity increased markedly and journal editors sought to manage the flood of submissions in a responsible way. In contemporary science, publication in a peer-reviewed (refereed) journal is the standard of accomplishment. But peer review has its critics, and some believe that it remains an open question if peer review really works. For the foreseeable future, peer review will continue as the process by which manuscripts are evaluated for publication. For all its faults, peer review does not appear to have a serious rival.

Authorship and Career Stages

First-authored papers carry substantial influence in the scientific community. For this reason, junior scientists should aspire to have at least some first-authored or sole-authored articles. Scientists who rarely or never have these kinds of authorships may find it difficult to demonstrate that they are capable of independent research. This problem is exacerbated when the junior scientist publishes exclusively with a mentor. Of course, authorship position should reflect scientific contribution, and a junior scientist should not expect that he or she will be given first authorship as a concession to career progress. It is unfortunately true that scientists who consistently appear far down the list of authors may not receive much recognition for their work, and sometimes will be virtually invisible in an *et al*. To be first or sole author carries a big advantage of visibility.

Junior scientists are well advised to develop a publication plan, taking into account the expected completion of research projects. Say, for example, that a scientist is involved in three projects, one of which would lead to a first-author publication while the other two would involve an author position that trails four or five other scientists. A strong case can be made to give primary effort to the paper on which the scientist would be first author, but, of course, without neglecting the other papers. We have known some highly capable junior scientists who, for one reason or another, do not publish sole- or first-authored papers. The lack of these kinds of authorship can be detrimental to promotion decisions and reviews of research grant applications. Obviously, then, it behooves a junior scientist to be as clear as possible about authorship on the projects with which he or she is connected. If the overall plan of research holds no prospect of a sole- or first-authored paper within a 5-year period, then it may be wise to reconsider the plan. Extenuating circumstances may apply, such as participation in team research and in which the investigator's role is clearly defined and deserves recognition. But exceptions are just that, deviations from the norm, and deviations require explanation and justification. A first-author paper stands on its own.

Selecting a Journal

It is advisable to decide where a paper will be submitted as early as possible in manuscript preparation. Journals have different style requirements, and they also differ in their target audience, limitations on manuscript length, types of manuscripts that will be considered, and other important factors. Although many scientists aspire to have a paper published in journals of highest impact (*Science, Nature, Proceedings of the National Academy of Sciences*), there is no shame in publishing exclusively in journals with lower impact factors. One consideration is the visibility of a paper in the thousands of articles that appear every month. It is estimated that about 40,000 scientific/engineering papers are published annually throughout the world, with about half of these being in biomedical journals (Brumback, 2009). How can any one article be noticed in this deluge of scientific information? One way is to ensure that the article is indexed in *Index Medicus* or its Internet-based successor *PubMed* (both are generated by the United States National Library of Medicine). *PubMed* includes about 5000 publications that have been judged to meet certain standards of publication quality. Articles appearing in these selected publications will be visible to those who search *PubMed*. These publications are not equal with respect to their perceived prestige or overall value. A further differentiation can be achieved by considering their impact value.

Impact Scores

Impact scores are designed to measure the influence of scientific journals and the articles that appear in them. Influence is determined primarily by the number of citations to articles published in a given journal, on the assumption that the more frequently cited articles are, the more important they are in shaping a field of science. Impact factors have been used for a number of purposes, including

1. Evaluating the scholarly value of a journal.

2. Ranking journals within a discipline.

3. Deciding journal cancellations or new purchases by a library system.

4. Providing guidance to a scientist on where to publish an article.

5. Assisting in evaluations for promotions, tenure decisions, project funding, and distribution of resources within an agency or institution.

6. Selecting journals to assist in a review of the literature on a particular topic.

The Web of Science (Institute for Scientific Information [ISI], from Thomson Reuters) covers more than 10,000 journals worldwide, including Open Access journals and over 110,000 conference proceedings. It offers coverage in the sciences, social sciences, arts, and humanities, extending to 1900. A part of the Web of Science, Journal Citation Reports (JCR), is designed to measure the influence and impact of research at both the journal and category levels. The basic idea underlying this index (and most efforts at calculating impact scores) is that impact is related to the number of times articles are cited. For example, the 2007 Impact Factor calculated by JCR for a journal is defined by the number of times articles published in the journal during 2005 to 2006 were cited in indexed journals during 2007. Several criticisms have been made of JCR, including:

1. The statistics are calculated for 2-year intervals (which may be too short to give a representative view).

2. The mean number of citations to papers published in a particular journal does not necessarily relate to the number of citations for a given paper in that journal.

3. The data do not include books, book chapters, dissertations, and non-ISI journals.

4. The database is biased toward English-language journals.

5. The disciplinary coverage is not uniform.

6. Citation behavior varies among disciplines.

7. The data includes self-citations.

8. A technical article will be highly cited even though the contribution is only on new procedures.

9. Poor quality articles may be cited frequently as authors refute their findings.

10. Subscription to the service is expensive.

There are several alternatives to the JCR Impact Factor. One is EigenFactor (http://www.eigenfactor.org/), which uses an algorithm similar to Google's PageRank (a link analysis algorithm that assigns a numerical weighting to each element of a hyperlinked set of documents). Compared to JCR, EigenFactor offers several advantages. It examines 5 years of data and includes non-ISI journals, books and dissertations. It also removes self-citations and determines a numerical score based not simply on number of citations but on citations by other influential journals. Another advantage is the cost—it is free.

SCImago Journal Rank (SJR) (http://www.scimagojr.com/), like Eigen-Factor, uses the PageRank algorithm and is free (http://www.scimagojr.com). It is based on Journals included in Scopus, a database that includes more than 13,000 journals and has more international diversity than the ISI database used by JCR. SJR analyzes 3 years of citations and removes self-citations. One limitation is that its citations go back only as far as about 1995.

Publish or Perish (PoP), based on Google Scholar citations, can calculate results by author or by journal. For the latter, it can analyze the average number of citations per paper, the average number of authors per paper, and the h-index (which combines an assessment of both quantity and quality of papers). Free software for PoP can be downloaded at http://www.harzing.com/pop.htm.

Finally, Stringer et al. (2008) describe a mathematical model that addresses two fundamental issues relating to the impact of a published scientific paper: (1) the time scale over which the impact of papers published in a given journal is fully expressed, and (2) the typical impact of papers published in a particular journal (Stringer, Sales-Pardo, & Nunes Amaral, 2008). Concerning the first issue, the authors found that the time over which full impact is demonstrated ranges from 1 to 26 years, depending on the journal. Computation of impact for periods of only 3 to 5 years obviously does a disservice to some fields. Concerning the second question, the authors determined that the papers in a given journal have a typical impact value and a well-defined range of impact value (Stringer et al., 2008).

Like peer review, impact scores have their faults. But they are likely to continue to be used for some time to come, so it is prudent for scientists to understand how they work and what their limitations are. One piece of advice is to consider several different scores, including the JCR Impact Factor, EigenFactor, SJR, and PoP, and to justify the selection based on considerations such as the field of science in which the contribution is made.

Writing for High-Impact Journals

As indicated earlier, the impact factor is calculated from data on the number of citations that a published article receives. This is a measure of influence, and not necessarily a measure of quality. To be sure, some research reports of very high quality probably would never be published in certain high-impact journals because they may not appeal to a general scientific audience (one of the primary criteria used by many high-impact journals). A scientist who wishes to submit to a journal with high impact should carefully study the instructions to contributors, examine recently published articles in that journal, and seek critical advice from others regarding their opinion of the importance and clarity of the report.

The Least Publishable Unit (LPU)

The least (or minimal) publishable unit is the smallest piece of a research project that has a likelihood of being published in a scientific journal. The notion of a LPU often is used in jest, but scientists do weigh various ways to publish their results and often for very good reason. If number of published articles is an accepted index of productivity, then trying to milk a project for as many publications as possible is sometimes taken as a strategy for career success. Taken to extremes, this strategy becomes ludicrous. There can be circumstances in which a single study, even a modest one, can result in two or more publications. For example, suppose that in preparing for a study, a scientist conducts a comprehensive review of a complex literature, distills the review into a succinct and effective summary of research, and identifies reasons for any discrepant findings. Such a review may be highly valuable, but if the scientist in question plans to submit a paper to a journal that considers only papers of limited length, the literature review may very well be sacrificed. The scientist can submit the literature review as a separate manuscript to another journal. Another example is the development and refinement of a laboratory technique that was successfully used in a series of studies. The technique may be sufficiently important that it becomes the subject of a manuscript submitted for publication. Generally obvious to reviewers and peer scientists is when authors set out to publish excessively from a single piece of research. Those who pursue this strategy will not add much to their reputations even if they succeed in adding to their lists of published articles.

A Final Word

It can be helpful to read general advice on scientific writing, and this chapter was written in that spirit. But writing is an obstacle to many scientists, and not only the junior ones. Writing is a craft, a skill. Good writing comes with practice and with careful attention to the writing of others with the intent of learning from their examples. Colleagues who are willing to read drafts of a paper can be a boon to the process, because they can point out ambiguities, logical errors, infelicities of wording, and other problems. Research has its primary influence through dissemination, and publication in scientific journals is the primary means to that end. It is important not only to learn the craft of scientific writing but also to become wise about peer review, impact factors, and other aspects of journal publishing.

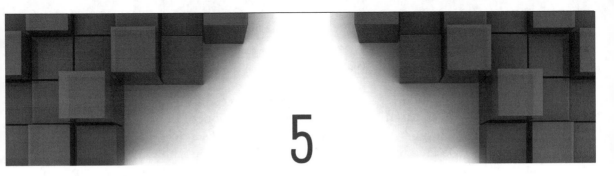

5

Membership in the Scientific Community

*T*he term "scientific community" is not an empty cliché. In fact, scientists are linked to one another in a variety of ways that strengthen the practice of science and contribute to career development and personal fulfillment. This chapter offers advice on how to become part of the scientific community and contribute to its vitality.

NETWORKING

Gone are the days (if they ever really existed) when science was a solitary enterprise in which individuals worked in relative isolation from their peers. Few scientists work that way now. Instead, scientists work in communities of specialists to share their work, support one another, form collaborations, ponder over problems, and obtain constructive criticism. Networking with colleagues can yield a variety of benefits, both tangible and intangible. It also takes a variety of forms, ranging from a casual face-to-face chat with a colleague over a cup of coffee to a group conversation with international participants held over the Internet. Ways to network are limited only by the creativity of those involved—and sometimes by budgetary constraints. Networking can be especially important in narrowly specialized areas of science where peer scientists are widely scattered. Particularly in small laboratories and universities, scientists may discover that there are no local colleagues who share their specialty.

The power of the Internet is being harnessed for networking. With this technology, an individual scientist can communicate with scientists in several different countries, exchanging information and opinions. Many different Web sites have been developed for specialty interests, so many that it is not possible to offer a current listing of these resources in this book. But a general purpose Web-based resource should be mentioned: the Community of Science (COS; http://www.cos.com) contains several services, including COS Expertise, COS Funding Opportunities, and COS Profile. The COS Expertise, a knowledge management system for individuals and institutions contains profiles for about 500,000 researchers from more than 1,600 institutions around the world. COS Funding Opportunities is said to be the world's most comprehensive funding resource, with more than 25,000 records that represent almost 400,000 opportunities. The COS Profile allows scientists to describe their research and expertise. It also includes a tool that can be used to maintain a current CV.

Networking is a tool to develop collaborations and enhance their effectiveness. Team science is growing rapidly and is fundamental to solving large and complex problems. In their analysis of team science, Wuchty, Jones, and Uzzi (2007) reviewed 19.9 million research articles over five decades and examined 2.1 million patents. The data were grouped in three main areas: science and engineering (171 subfields), social sciences (54 subfields), and arts and humanities (27 subfields). The results indicated that teams increasingly dominate in knowledge production, and a strong shift toward collective research was evident in science and engineering, social sciences, and patents. A smaller shift was seen in the arts and humanities. In each area, work by teams dominated the top of the citation distribution. This transition to team science affects the way in which research is conceived and performed, while redefining the roles of individual scientists. Team science can create opportunities that would not emerge from the work of an individual scientist working alone, but it carries with it a pattern of responsibility to the group as a whole. Team science also transcends some traditional boundaries. Jones et al. (2008) reported that multi-university collaborations are the most rapidly growing type of authorship structure and they produce the highest impact papers when a top-tier university is included (B. F. Jones, Wuchty, & Uzzi, 2008).

But, having said all this, we hasten to add that scientists should not despair just because they are not currently part of a team or are not affiliated with an elite university. The history of science is replete with stories of scientists working alone or with a colleague or two who make exciting discoveries. Science still moves ahead largely because someone hatches an idea and pursues it. Intuition and innovation are not necessarily products of a team. And for those who desire team membership, it is good to remember that individual contributions to science may pave the way to becoming a member of a team.

REVIEWING FOR JOURNALS

Peer review is one of the aspects of scientific writing and publishing covered in Chapter 4, but the intent of the discussion in this chapter is to examine how scientists participate in peer review as one of their professional activities. Reviewing for journals is a responsibility that scientists share to ensure that the peer review process effectively accomplishes its goal of ensuring the credibility of scientific reports. Quite simply, reviewing papers that have been submitted to scientific journals is part of the life of a scientist. This is not to say that one should necessarily accept every request for a manuscript review, but rather that one should expect to review a certain number of papers in a year and should devote the time needed for a thoughtful evaluation. Reviews should be taken very seriously, because they are an essential part of the process of science.

Reviewing papers submitted to journals can pay dividends in the form of increased knowledge about a topic, a better appreciation of scientific techniques, an exposure to a new area of scientific study, and practice in critical thinking. Employers sometimes recognize the importance of manuscript reviews in their performance evaluations. This is particularly true of universities. For this reason, it is wise to keep a record of the journals for which manuscript reviews have been submitted.

The following are pointers for someone who is new to the process of peer review for scientific journals.

It is wise to read carefully the instructions to reviewers and the purpose of the journal in question. Although all scientific journals are concerned with the merit of a research paper, they may differ in the importance assigned to relevance of the topic, the general versus narrow interest of the paper, and the length of the report. Often, a paper that is rejected by one journal is accepted by another, and not simply because one journal is more demanding of scientific quality. Journals that appeal to a wide readership may reject a very good paper because it is not considered to have broad interest. And, to take the opposite situation, a very good overview paper may be rejected because the journal is devoted to fresh empirical research.

The following suggestions pertain to the reviewer's role:

1. Be respectful. Reviews can be bluntly critical without being personally offensive. The authors of this book know of promising young scientists who were gravely disheartened by a review that was unnecessarily harsh.

2. Honor due dates for reviews. If you cannot possibly complete the review within the requested date, contact the editor and indicate when you will be able to submit the review. Egregious delays have occurred because reviewers fail to submit their comments in a timely manner. These delays can be frustrating to the editor and the contributor (who often blames the journal for the slow editorial process).

3. Remember that, for almost all journals, a submitted manuscript is considered confidential and is for assigned reviewers' eyes only during the review process. If you want to consult a colleague, first obtain permission from the editor. If you are inclined to ask a graduate student or postdoctoral fellow to read the paper as part of their training, do not do so unless you have received permission from the editor. Do not leave the contributed

manuscript on a shelf in the laboratory, on a table in the lounge, or in some other public place. It is your responsibility to guard the manuscript and keep its contents private. This injunction also bars the reviewer from discussing the paper with a colleague or mentioning it in a lecture or other event. If you have a printed copy of the manuscript, destroy it when the review is complete. If you have saved an electronic copy on your computer, delete the file. Retaining your review comments until the editorial decision is made is acceptable and advisable, if only to have a backup copy in case the submitted review is lost.

4. Be as constructive as possible. A flawed manuscript often can be saved with advice from reviewers. It is not your task to rewrite the paper, but if you have suggestions that can substantially improve the science, be sure to offer them. Competent reviewers have a major role in making science a powerful tool for understanding. Frequently, it is helpful to support review comments with citations of relevant literature. Such reference authenticates the comments.

5. If a manuscript is marred by numerous errors in grammar, word choice, and style, you do not need to correct every instance. Simply mention in your review that the paper needs to be reworked to remedy these problems.

6. Always be conscious of a possible conflict of interest. One facet of this conflict is if the paper in question criticizes or rejects a theory that you have espoused. So long as the data are valid and the interpretation is reasonable, the author has the right to develop the paper as he or she sees fit.

7. If a possible issue of research misconduct is noticed, it should not be ignored. The integrity of science depends on the vigilance of all concerned, and reviewers definitely have a role in detecting ethical breaches.

8. Many journals will advise the reviewers of the editorial decision on a submitted manuscript and often will include copies of the reviews. This is an excellent learning opportunity because you can compare your responses with those of your peers.

STUDY SECTIONS AND REVIEW PANELS

Government and private agencies generally rely on peer review to help determine the scientific merit of applications for research grants and contracts. Experts usually are selected for assistance in peer review based on their publications, funding, and overall reputation. An invitation to serve on study sections and review panels is an honor, but it also can be a lot of work for little or no monetary compensation. Many scientists agree to this service because they believe they should "pay their dues" by participating in the peer-review process. There is return for this service because it offers an unparalleled opportunity to see the cutting edge of science in the form of fresh research questions and innovative methods.

Reviewing research applications is similar in some respects to reviewing manuscripts submitted for publication, but it also differs in important ways. The similarities pertain to the general ways of doing science, including careful scholarship, carefully chosen research design, and consideration of risks to the research. But a major difference is that the research paper is a complete report on a study or experiment, whereas the research application is a design for research. The reviewer must decide on the likelihood of a valuable outcome from the proposed research.

Review panels convene in face-to-face meetings, teleconferences, or Web-based discussions. Given that face-to-face meetings are relatively costly because of expenses for transportation, lodging, and meals, funding agencies often look to other means of assembling expert opinion. Teleconferences are much less expensive and retain much of the verbal exchange of a face-to-face meeting. Web-based technologies for hosting meetings are changing rapidly and offer several advantages that may make them increasingly attractive. Whatever the mode of convening the reviewers, the meeting typically is led by a chair, who generally is selected from members in the group of reviewers. The chair has the responsibility of keeping the discussion on track and summarizing major points of agreement or disagreement.

Reviewers may be standing members of a panel or committee, but others may be ad hoc reviewers who are called on to assist in the reviews on a limited-term basis. In the NIH Center for Scientific Review (CSR) system, study section members usually are appointed to 4-year terms. At the time of the writing of this book, the CSR Web site described the selection of reviewers in terms of four main categories of requirements: General, Expertise, Study-Section Specific, and Individual Qualifications. In terms of general requirements, suitable candidates are recognized authorities in their field, principal investigators on a research project comparable to those under review, and must be dedicated to reviews that are fair and of high quality. In addition, members are selected to ensure diversity with respect to geographic distribution, gender, race, and ethnicity. Expertise requirements are determined by the scientific areas under review, including the need to ensure coverage of emerging areas of science and shifting scientific boundaries.

CONDUCT AT MEETINGS

As obvious as it may sound, personal behavior at meetings should be courteous, considerate, and professional. Inevitably, scientists come under the judgment of their colleagues in any setting in which science is at stake. This is not to say that scientists are inherently judgmental, but only to note that issues of trust and reliability are constants in science and those who practice it. An ill-considered offhand remark can have its consequences. Scientific meetings are opportunities to prove your worth as a scientist. The ideal pattern of conduct is to preserve collegiality and mutual esteem while weighing the scientific merit of a research proposal, an idea, or other intellectual product.

Professional competence can be shown without indulging in pedantry, vicious criticism of other scientists, and disdain for other ways of doing things. One vital lesson that most scientists learn is that they can be, and often are, wrong. The conceit of always being right is a hindrance to science, especially when a scientist clings to a theory or conclusion that is eroded by mounting counterevidence. Data should always trump passion when it comes to a particular theory or long-held belief. Reason and appeal to evidence are the bywords of a fruitful discussion. Egos should be checked at the door, not stroked in the meeting room.

WRITING LETTERS OF RECOMMENDATION

Peer review is a standard for much of the work in science. It is the basic means for determining the merit of applications for research support and the merit of manuscripts submitted for publication. It also is the standard way of evaluating the competence and performance of individual scientists, for the purposes of employment, contract extension, promotion, or special recognition (e.g., awards). It is customary for organizations that employ scientists to seek external evaluations for all of the purposes just noted. These evaluations take the form of a letter of appraisal that speaks to a scientist's professional accomplishments or the potential for such accomplishments. An invitation to participate in the evaluation of a colleague's scholarly achievements is an honor itself, because it shows that the requesting individual or agency respects your opinion and believes that it should carry weight in the decision process.

Letters of recommendation are central to career advancement, but it is unfortunately rare that a scientist would have received any advice or training on how to prepare such letters. From our experience, it is clear that some well-intended letter writers fail to serve their purpose. Therefore, we offer a few guidelines on how to prepare a letter. These guidelines are general in nature and would necessarily be refined for a particular purpose. For example, a letter that endorses a prospective employee is not the same as a letter that supports promotion to a senior rank within an organization.

1. Review the criteria established by the organization. Agencies often have established criteria for hiring, retaining, or promoting an individual scientist. The letter of recommendation should acknowledge these criteria. Avoid the "form letter" approach in which comments are cast in the broadest possible terms with no reference to the qualifications for the position in question.

2. The organization may send a set of materials to be considered in the external evaluation. These materials may include any or all of the following: a curriculum vitae (or resume), a statement of the individual's research plan, a record of external and internal research support, selected reprints, teaching evaluations, and other items pertinent to the position in question. The letter writer should review these materials and be prepared to mention them in the letter. By "mention" we mean a thoughtful consideration of their importance. It can be particularly helpful to comment on how individual papers influenced a line of research or resolved a long-standing controversy.

3. You may be asked to rank the individual compared to others of comparable experience and responsibility. Such rankings can be difficult but they are helpful to the employing institution because they go beyond general descriptors.

4. The letter should be a fair and honest appraisal, free of hyperbole and gratuitous flattery. Peer review demands a conscientious effort to identify the individual's career accomplishments (or potential) and to document the evaluation with appropriate reference to publications, professional activity, and awards. Even senior professionals sometimes submit a letter that is nearly vacuous and amounts to little more than noise in the system.

5. If the person or persons issuing the request for an evaluation ask for your opinion in an area in which you lack sufficient information or expertise, it is better to decline comment than to fabricate a judgment.

PROFESSIONAL ORGANIZATIONS

Scientists generally find that one or more professional organizations are closely aligned with their interests. These organizations provide networking opportunities and many other types of support. Not surprisingly, many scientists feel an obligation to a professional organization and volunteer to serve as an officer, committee member, or in other ways that promote the organization. Not everyone will, or should, become deeply involved in professional leadership but each member of an organization should accept the responsibility for prompt payment of dues, responding to relevant surveys or inquiries, and participating when possible in functions such as annual meetings. One reason to do so is to network with colleagues in a specialty area. Another is that professional organizations can achieve by their number of members what a single individual can rarely do. On occasion, the influence of a professional society can be profound, for example, by affecting public policy, by promoting a practice that is widely beneficial, or by eliminating a practice that has unintended ill effects.

In general, professional societies are not wealthy organizations. Much of the operational revenue is derived from dues that are paid for the privilege of membership. Many societies develop nondues revenue streams by selling products or services, but even then, the total operations budget is usually modest. Professional societies often accomplish much more than might be expected from the size of their annual budgets because members of the society freely give their expertise and labor for the greater causes that the organization represents. It is the intellectual, rather than the financial, resources of the organization that really matter.

Science-wide organizations are considered in the next section.

WHO SPEAKS FOR THE SCIENTIFIC COMMUNITY?

With the exception of specialty organizations, the community of scientists is a very loose organization whose membership is more implicit than explicit. Those who most readily identify with the scientific community have advanced degrees (PhD or equivalent) and an affiliation with an academic or research institution. There is no membership card, no voting forum, and no board of directors. Given this flexibility, it might well be asked how the community can be influential outside its own ranks of specialists? Is there a voice for science in the broadest sense?

Some entities have a fairly strong voice in speaking on behalf of science. They include the American Association for the Advancement of Science (AAAS), Sigma Xi, and the National Academies. The last consists of the National Academy of Sciences (NAS), the National Academy of Engineering (NAE), the Institute of Medicine (IOM), and the National Research Council (NRC).

According to its Web site (http://www.aaas.org/) AAAS is:

> An international nonprofit organization dedicated to advancing science around the world by serving as an educator, leader, spokesperson, and professional association. In addition to organizing membership activities, AAAS publishes the journal *Science* as well as many scientific newsletters, books and reports, and spearheads programs that raise the bar of understanding for science worldwide.

Reading *Science* can be very helpful in keeping up with recent developments across science as a whole.

Sigma Xi is the international honor society of science and engineering. It has 60,000 members who were elected to membership based on their research potential or achievements. The Sigma Xi Web site (http://www.sigmaxi.org/) notes that, "More than 500 Sigma Xi chapters in North America and around the world provide a supportive environment for interdisciplinary research at colleges and universities, industry research centers and government laboratories." Sigma XI publishes the *American Scientist* magazine and provides grants-in-aid-of-research for undergraduate and graduate students. It supports surveys such as the survey of postdoctoral fellows which is discussed in more detail in Chapter 10 (Davis, 2005).

Turning now to the National Academies, including the National Academy of Sciences (NAS), National Academy of Engineering (NAE), Institute of Medicine (IOM), and the National Research Council (NRC), the NAS is "an honorific society of distinguished scholars engaged in scientific and engineering research, dedicated to the furtherance of science and technology and to their use for the general welfare." Its membership numbers about 2,100 individuals along with about 380 foreign affiliates. The NAE, which provides engineering leadership in service to the nation, has more than 2,000 peer-elected members and foreign associates. The IOM Web site (http://www.iom.edu/) describes its mission as follows:

> The Institute provides a vital service by working outside the framework of government to ensure scientifically informed analysis and independent guidance. The IOM's mission is to serve as adviser to the nation to improve health. The IOM provides unbiased, evidence-based, and authoritative information and advice concerning health and science policy to policy-makers, professionals, leaders in every sector of society, and the public at large.

The NRC, which functions under the auspices of the NAS, NAE, and IOM, has its mission "to improve government decision making and public policy, increase public education and understanding, and promote the acquisition and dissemination of knowledge in matters involving science, engineering, technology, and health." Approximately 6,000 scientists, engineers, and professionals volunteer to accomplish this mission.

Some of these organizations are mentioned elsewhere in this book as they pertain to particular issues. For example, the Institute of Medicine published the report, *Beyond the HIPAA Privacy Rule: Enhancing Privacy, Improving Health Through Research*. Among the publications of the NRC is *Research Doctorate Programs in the United States: Continuity and Change*, which is a detailed analysis of the status of research doctorate programs, along with recommendations for improvements. Through its numerous publications (over 200 annually), the NRC is a world leader in the dissemination of free scientific information, most of which is available at http://www.nap.edu.

BEING SELECTIVE

A scientist's plate can easily fill to the point of overextending time and energy. Even for individuals who do not have teaching or administrative responsibilities, there are many aspects of a career in science that can consume effort. In this chapter, we have considered a few of the activities that are part of a scientist's schedule. Although it may be tempting for junior scientists to say yes to every request for a manuscript review, service on a study section or review panel, or helping with a professional organization, these tasks come with the possibility of overcommitment and personal stress. It is prudent to weigh these opportunities carefully and be sure that they do not become so demanding of effort that one's own research and essential obligations are pushed aside. When an external request for assistance comes at a bad time (such as shortly before the deadline for a current grant application), it is perfectly acceptable to decline, but do so promptly and politely. It is wise to leave the door open for future requests, unless you have a particular reason to discourage a person or agency from contacting you again.

Availability also is affected by life situations, such as beginning a new position, maternity leave, child-care responsibilities, administrative or committee workload, developing a laboratory, or newly developed research collaboration. It is important to set priorities and apply them to schedules and to new developments.

All opportunities are not equal. Certain professional activities carry higher prestige, more opportunities for networking, or better possibilities for learning. For example, serving as a member of the editorial board of one journal may be preferable to serving as an anonymous reviewer for another journal. Some committees offer higher visibility than others. Some consulting arrangements can offer long-term advantages in career development. It may seem crass to speak of career development, but scientists are not immune from planning for their careers, and current trends make career planning even more critical. The rapid growth of team science, the high cost of developing and maintaining laboratories, the need for creativity and flexibility in obtaining funding—all place a premium on planning for career development.

COPING WITH CONFLICT, REJECTION, AND UNCERTAINTY

An honest appraisal of the life of scientists must acknowledge that there will be times of conflict, rejection, and uncertainty. Conflicts may arise because of disagreements about selecting a research method, determining order of authorship, hiring or dismissing a member of the research staff, or dealing with an ethical problem. Some colleagues may seem arrogant and unwilling to compromise, so that resolution of a problem demands great patience. Rejection takes several forms, but the ones of greatest impact are rejection of a paper submitted to a journal, failure to obtain funding for a research project, a negative decision on promotion or tenure, failure to obtain a desired work position, and loss of resources needed for research. Resilience is necessary to withstand these rejections and to continue with career plans (possibly revised). Uncertainty about research project funding, promotion to tenure, and publications can result in stress and anxiety. Even senior scientists with many years of continuous extramural support for their research find that a research application has not been selected for funding, placing into jeopardy a long-standing research laboratory.

These circumstances can be trying, but it may help to know that all scientists face unpleasant circumstances at some point in their careers. It should never be assumed that scientists are isolated from the vagaries of life, and it should always be remembered that rejection is not the same thing as failure. There can be much truth in the reflection, "It was not a failure, but a learning experience." In the highly competitive world of contemporary science, there probably will be several qualified applicants for a professional position, there will be more meritorious research grant applications than there is money to support them, and more high-quality manuscripts submitted to a high-impact journal than there are pages to publish all of them. One scientist said the following about research grant applications: "If you are not getting rejections, you are not submitting grant applications."

CONCLUSION

One of the most satisfying aspects of a career in science is working in an arena populated by colleagues who are driven by a pursuit of knowledge. And even as they might compete with one another for resources and prestige, they are inevitably linked in a system of peer reviews that enjoins them to place ideas above personalities. Interactions with scientific colleagues contribute to personal fulfillment and professional maturation.

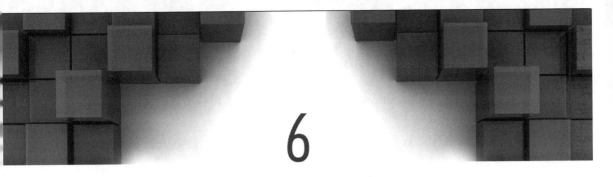

6

Good Research Practices

Good research practices (GRP) training has received increasing attention within the scientific community. Most often scientists learn research practices during their research training based on the practices used in the laboratory or group where they train. As a result, although it is agreed that careful documentation and data management are required for conducting research, few resources provide detailed directions on how this should be done.

There are detailed guidelines for laboratories developing food additives and drug development that were developed by the Food and Drug Administration and published in 2005 (http://www.nal.usda.gov/awic/legislat/21cfr 97.htm) in the *Federal Register*. These do not apply, however, to basic research. At present, there are not universally accepted guidelines for documenting research, although there are generally accepted practices required for research.

Clinical research, however, is more standardized, and good clinical practice (GCP) refers to international standards that provide quality controls and ethical standards for research involving humans and patients in particular. These have become relatively well formulated (International Conference on Harmonisation, 1997).

Good research practices are important to follow at each stage of research, including: initial meetings to design a study, authorship discussions, development of the research procedures, designing checklists and case reports, documentation of procedures and data acquisition, data analysis, manuscript development and revisions, and submission and revision for publication. The basis for following good research practices are to:

1. Keep track of what was done to prevent errors in recapitulation of the conduct of the research, particularly at the manuscript writing stage;

2. Document authorship decisions and the basis for any changes in authorship during the conduct of the research;

3. Document the role of each of the authors in the research, which many journals now require be reported:

   a. who was involved in the conceptualization of the research,

   b. who designed the procedures, conducted the research,

   c. who was involved in data analysis, and

   d. who participated in writing the manuscript?

4. Provide evidence of inventorship in the event of the development of any intellectual property during the conduct of the research;

5. Maintain adequate documentation in the event of a research audit; and

6. In the case of clinical research, maintain adequate documentation of each of the research participants in the event of an audit by the Institutional Review Board (IRB).

Throughout the research process, all events should be tracked, usually in a laboratory notebook (Figure 6–1). The same functions are now being performed using electronic laboratory notebooks (ELN) that conform to documentation requirements for both intellectual property and to meet FDA requirements GCP for clinical trials. Many pharmacologic companies now use these systems although universities and research institutions have been slow to adopt these systems, most likely because of cost and training requirements.

OFFICE OF RESEARCH INTEGRITY OF THE U.S. DEPARTMENT OF HEALTH AND HUMAN SERVICES

The vast majority of scientists are honest, hard working, and careful in their research practices. However, a small percentage commit scientific misconduct; that is, either they plagiarize others' work, fabricate results, or falsify research. Given the importance of science to society, its support by taxpayer funds, and its' importance to patient care, scientific misconduct is a major concern. The most egregious cases often appear in the lay press. As a result of past and current cases, formal processes have been developed for reporting, investigating, and administering penalties for scientific misconduct.

The Office of Research Integrity (ORI) is an independent office within the Department of Health and Human Services in the United States. All institutions receiving federal research funds are under obligation to monitor research integrity, support a confidential reporting system, investigate meaningful charges, and report the results of internal investigations to the ORI. If suspected misconduct is reported by the institution to the ORI, the ORI may

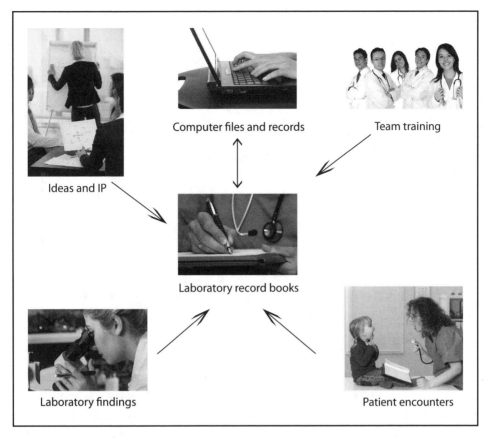

Computer files and records

Team training

Ideas and IP

Laboratory record books

Laboratory findings

Patient encounters

FIGURE 6–1. Aspects of the research process, such as team training, patient encounters, and laboratory findings should be tracked in a laboratory notebook or using research documentation software known as Electronic Laboratory Notebooks (ELN). Images from Shutterstock® All rights reserved.

further investigate the case, come to a conclusion, and decide on whether disciplinary actions apply (Figure 6-2).

The ORI provides excellent research training materials. The Introduction to the Responsible Conduct of Research is an overview of good research practices (http://ori.dhhs.gov/documents/rcrintro.pdf). In addition, the ORI publishes a quarterly newsletter which is available in electronic form from the ORI homepage (http://ori.hhs.gov) as well as a listing of both face to face courses and Web-based training materials. The best way to prevent research misconduct is to ensure training on responsible research conduct, which has increased in emphasis at most institutions over recent years.

A scientist may not be guilty of misconduct but a charge may be alleged against them (see Figure 6-2). This can result in the institution retrieving and securing all records of the research in order to investigate the allegations, and can cause a major disruption in the laboratory in addition to considerable

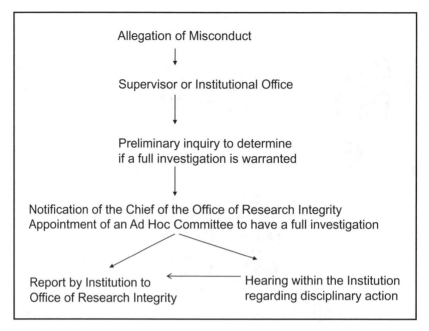

FIGURE 6–2. Process of investigation of research misconduct.

stress. In some cases, no intentional misconduct has occurred but the investigator and their team may not have used adequate documentation during the research processes to demonstrate that the data was accurately recorded, processed, and analyzed before publication. In such cases, the investigation and deliberation process can be long and painful. Therefore, following good research practices is important when documenting a study to address any questions that may arise at any time during or for several years following the publication of research.

LABORATORY NOTEBOOKS

The traditional way of documenting research is to use bound notebooks, preferably with the pages numbered. All entries should be in ink and dated. Discussions among members of the team should list who was present, and if intellectual property is involved, it may be important to have each person present to initial and date next to their name. No pages can be removed and any empty or erroneous entries should be crossed out but not erased and the reasons for crossing out documentation should be provided and dated. Empty pages usually have a diagonal line drawn across them with "empty page" written along the line.

During the research design process, after the initial questions and hypotheses are identified, procedures and outcome variables are identified; the research team should design the data management process. Before human research can begin, it must be reviewed and approved by the Institutional Review Board (IRB) designated by the U.S. Department of Health and Human Services by granting an institutional assurance. In the case of animal research, the Institutional Animal Care and Use Committee (IACUC) must review and approve the research protocol. If a human research protocol or an animal protocol covers the research, care should be taken to make certain at each stage that the research is in compliance with the protocol. If changes are needed, amendments should be submitted to the IRB or IACUC and the research put on hold until the amendment is approved.

Laboratory books should not leave the laboratory to prevent loss; they are the property of the institution and must remain there until they can be destroyed using proper procedures; no earlier than 5 years, and usually 7 years after publication. Students and other members of the investigative team can be given permission to take copies their laboratory books with them when they leave, particularly if they are still writing up the research.

ELECTRONIC LABORATORY NOTEBOOK SOFTWARE (ELN)

In recent years we have seen a rapid expansion of the development of electronic record keeping replacing the pen and ink laboratory notebook with e-notebooks (Butler, 2005). Some ELNs are very expensive and need to be subscribed to by institutions; many were developed for large commercial labs supported by pharmacological companies. LABtrack is one example (http://www.labtrack.com) but is now available for small laboratories at a more reasonable cost (approximately $1,500 per year for a team of 10 or less after the initial subscription cost, which is usually over $10,000). This software can use an Oracle database, which is an accepted standard for Food and Drug Administration monitored research. That is, it keeps track of every data entry and who was involved in any data changes which is required for tracking clinical research databases. NoteBookMaker is less expensive, particularly for academia, but depends on Filemaker Pro for use on a Network (http://www.notebook maker.com/store/page17/page17.html) . SigmaCERF is another product that meets good research practices and intellectual property documentation standards and FDA requirements for good clinical practice (http://www.sigma plot.com/products/SIGMA_CERF/index.php). For clinical research, Oracle is a standard (http://www.oracle.com/webapps/dialogue/dlgpage.jsp?p_ext=Y&p_dlg_id=8235024&src=6712278&Act=48&sckw=WWHS08106311MPP068 .GCM.8340.150) and is used for a large percentage of large multi-institutional clinical trials, but can be expensive.

For the small academic laboratory involved in basic research, eCAT, developed by Axiope Limited (http://www.axiope.com/electronic_lab_note book_faq.html) was recently introduced at a reasonable price and is fully Web-based, allowing members of a laboratory group to share information from anywhere (approximate cost is the same for a team of 10, about $1,500 per year).

This is a rapidly changing field and only a small percentage of academic laboratories are using this software, estimated at about 8% in 2005 (Butler, 2005), but that is likely to change in the near future as research becomes more complex and the legal demands for tracking clinical trials and filing patents become better met by electronic notebooks than the old paper-based system. A significant advantage of ELNs over laboratory notebooks is that they prevent the loss of information, tracking of the research process is centralized, and physical storage space is not a problem. The disadvantages are cost and the need for training of all individuals in the laboratory.

Checklists

For many experiments, once the procedures are decided on it is best to follow checklists each time the procedure is run. The checklist can be stapled into the laboratory book or done on the computer and the name and location of the file entered into the laboratory book. File management software programs also can be used but must be saved and backed up and their existence and location documented in the lab book. Loose papers are a risk as they can easily be lost or misplaced; scanning papers and storing them as ".pdf" files and documenting them in the lab book can prevent the loss of loose papers or checklists.

Checklists are recommended as a way of documenting the research, maintaining quality, and preventing errors. They can include checks for setup and calibration of equipment, recording calibration values, recording monitoring values for in vivo studies, listing samples and vial numbers, and to ensure that each step of the research was followed in the same way. These can be part of an ELN documentation system.

Protecting Participants' Identities

Making human samples anonymous is now essential for protection of participant confidentiality. Sequential numbers should be assigned as soon as a participant is consented into a protocol. A master list of patient identifiers and their assigned numbers should be locked in a secure file cabinet. Participant data records based on assigned numbers should be kept on a secure server that is compliant with The Health Insurance Portability and Accountability Act of 1996 (HIPAA) Privacy and Security Rules (http://www.hhs.gov/ocr/privacy). Using sequential numbers ensures that only the IRB-approved number of participants in each group are admitted to a protocol. Laptops and other movable storage (flash drives) should not contain participant identifiers such as names or hospital numbers; only the anonymous sequential participant numbers should be included on movable storage.

Documentation of Data Processing

Data processing and analysis should be documented either in a word file (noted in the lab book) or written in the ELN record. The versions of the data at each step of the process should be retained so that all of the steps can be reviewed for errors or in the case of an audit. Each member of the research team must be alert to potential errors in the research such as:

1. Loss of the master list of subjects

2. Loss of group codes for identifying treatment group

3. Documentation of any changes in procedures

4. Documentation of all data processing or changes in the data

5. Decisions made by the research team during the conduct of the research and a check that these conformed to the IRB or ACUC approved protocol.

Training All Members of a Research Team

Students and new laboratory members must be trained on using good research practices. As different practices may be used by different investigators, new persons to the laboratory should be oriented on good research practices and how these are being following within the laboratory. A manual of standard operating procedures should be made available to all laboratory newcomers. Often, a checklist of training courses on animal procedures, IRB regulations, good research practices, should be completed by new arrivals to a laboratory. This should be reviewed by the principal investigator to make certain the new arrival has completed the necessary training before beginning research. To ensure that they are documenting and following the approved research protocol and procedures, there must be a regular review of their laboratory book or entries in the ELN, particularly when beginning to ensure that documentation is complete and accurate so that others could reconstruct the entire research project.

PREVENTION OF SCIENTIFIC MISCONDUCT

Scientific misconduct can sometimes happen inadvertently. Persons in the research team may be reading previous papers published by others or in the laboratory, IRB, or ACUC research protocols, and grant applications. Great care must be taken not to copy others' work unless it was previously published and must be attributed to the original work by citation.

Often, people collaborate and share research protocols, serve as grant reviewers or review manuscripts for journals. Grant proposals and journal articles under review are confidential; once the review is complete, they should not be kept on a persons' hard drive if they have not been published or are not in the public domain. Others' unpublished research must be protected and attributed to the original author if cited as "personal correspondence," as long as the person who is the source has given permission. If a data set was already published, any further publication of data from the same experiment, such as controls for comparisons for patients, must be cited in the methods section; otherwise, it is misleading to suggest that these were new data collected for the study. This is the only way in which the same data can be published more than once; all subsequent manuscripts must describe what portion of the data were already published and cite the previous publications. Otherwise, it is not ethical to publish the same data set twice or different data gathered from the same participants. A scientist is committing misconduct without citing any previous publication of the data from subjects that was previously published; publication of the same dataset without clear citation is considered falsification.

Misrepresentations represent falsification of the study and the data analysis. For example, if several variables were measured during the study and tested for significance but only the significant results are presented in the publication, this represents falsification. The fact that other work was done as part of the study and was not reported or mentioned in the manuscript is inaccurate. Rather, the manuscript should mention that the other data collected did not show significant results and are not being presented. The reviewers can then decide whether the full results should be presented.

Fabrication of research results is clearly scientific misconduct. Care must also be taken when doing figures that no changes in the data are made that might be considered falsification or fabrication. Alteration in graphs or photographs is considered misconduct and is prohibited.

HUMAN SUBJECTS PROTECTION FROM RESEARCH RISKS

The first responsibility of the research scientist involved in clinical research using human beings is to do no harm; that is, that participants should not experience adverse consequences as a result of the research. Any expected discomfort or short-term decrement in function that may occur and was approved by the IRB for inclusion in the research must be described to the participants before they agree to participate. Participation must be voluntary and the participants must be fully informed of the possible risks and benefits from participating in the research. When the participants in a research study may not benefit; the objective should be to benefit persons in general by doing research that will improve the diagnosis, treatment, or prevention of a disease or disorder. As such, the research should be relevant to others with the disease or disorder.

Irresponsible conduct in clinical research can put participants at risk for harm and result in the loss of society's trust in the clinical research enterprise. History, both recent and past, provides us with examples of irresponsible conduct in clinical research, some intentional and some unintentional (Francis, 2001). Although many examples of drug side effects or surgical outcomes that were unexpected or not explained to patients make the lay press, behavioral intervention can also involve risk. One example was a 1939 study that examined the effects of diagnostic labeling and frequent speech correction on speech fluency in six normally speaking children (Silverman, 1988). The intervention may have increased the risk of a chronic lifelong stuttering problem in those who were participants without their informed consent. Another is the Tuskegee experiment in the 1950s where investigators intentionally withheld treatment from participants in a study on the natural progression of untreated syphilis. Both of these are clearly unethical treatment of human participants in research, and violated the most important ethical responsibility of a clinical investigator—to prevent harm to research participants.

INSTITUTIONAL REVIEW BOARD OR ETHICS BOARD

In 1976, a conference was held for four days to address the ethical principles of research with human subjects. The result was the Belmont Report, which is the foundation for current practices of human protections during participation in research (http://ohsr.od.nih.gov/guidelines/belmont.html). This document addresses some underlying principles such as: (1) respect for persons as autonomous individuals, (2) beneficence by protecting persons from harm and securing their well-being while respecting their decisions, and (3) assuring justice in allowing fairness in allowing access to the benefits of research. It also outlines each of the components of research: (1) Informed consent providing information, comprehension, voluntariness; (2) assessment of risks and benefits; and (3) selection of subjects.

Research with human subjects can be justified on the basis that it will be of benefit to the society at large. This requires, therefore, that the research is well designed and valid so that it can provide significant new information to address a societal need. More important, however, is the safeguard of the participants' rights and protection from harm by the investigator and the research team. This is assured through prior review of the research plan by the Institutional Review Board (IRB) or Ethics Board composed of scientific peers, ethicists, and lay persons. The IRB then entrusts the principal investigator (PI) and the research team with protecting the participants from harm by following the approved research plan and reporting back to the IRB any observations of unexpected or adverse events that might indicate an increase in the risk of harm to the participants. Regulations of clinical research are aimed at: (1) providing increased assurances that participants in research are fully informed of all potential risks and benefits, and (2) assuring that the participants are not harmed by participating in the research, particularly when they are normal volunteers (World Medical Association, October 2000).

Several documents apply to clinical research:

1. Title 45 Code of Federal Regulations Part 46 entitled "Protection of Human Subjects" Revised June 18, 1991 and effective August 19, 1991 is available at: http://ohsr.od.nih.gov/guidelines/45cfr46.html (Title 45 Code of Federal Regulations Part 46, 1991). This is referred to as 45 CFR 46 and contains the federal regulations that apply to federally funded clinical research involving human participants.

2. The 1997 International Committee on Harmonization (ICH), has issued guidelines for clinical research on what would be considered good clinical practice (GCP) (International Conference on Harmonisation, 1997). The ICH Guidelines and topics are reviewed in the *Federal Register*, Vol. 62, No. 242, p. 66113, Wednesday, December 17, 1997. Most of these are available through the Food and Drug Administration Web site, http://www.fda.gov.

3. *The Trial Investigator's GCP Handbook: A Practical Guide To ICH Requirements* 2nd Edition by David Hutchinson, Brookwood Medical Publications, Brookwood, Surray, UK.

4. *The Declaration of Helsinki*, 2000, which addressed the need for further protection of research participants from harm and recommended limiting the use of placebos in clinical research to when there are no known or established effective treatments available for the disorder being studied (Food and Drug Administration, 1999; World Medical Association, October 2000).

5. "What makes clinical research ethical" by E. Emanual et al. was also used in the development of this chapter (Emanuel, Wendler, & Grady, 2000).

Because regulations governing clinical research often change, clinical investigators need to become knowledgeable in this area as part of their research training. Such investigators and students should be familiar with the documents cited above. Also recommended are the "Standards for Clinical Research within the NIH Intramural Research Program" available at http://www.cc.nih.gov/ccc/clinicalresearch/standards.html . Clinical investigators at medical research institutions are now required to receive training annually in this area. This chapter provides only a general overview of responsible practices in clinical research at the present time.

WHEN IS IT ETHICAL TO CONDUCT RESEARCH WITH HUMAN SUBJECTS?

Emanual et al. (2000) provided seven ethical requirements for research with human subjects:

1. The planned study must have social or scientific value. The research should have potential for either improved knowledge of diseases or disorders or developing more effective treatments for diseases or disorders.

2. The study must have scientific validity. A study must be well designed to ensure that the data will be adequate to answer the research question, and therefore, of use to others in society.

3. Participant selection must be fair and equitable. Efforts should be made to ensure that participants are not excluded on the basis of gender, age, or ethnic origin unless relevant to the disorder under study.

4. There must be a favorable risk-benefit ratio. If there is a risk of harm to participants, this must be balanced by potential benefit for the same participants.

5. The research is reviewed by an independent committee of peers, ethicists, and lay persons, usually the IRB or Ethics Board.

6. The informed consent of participants will ensure that they know and understand what is being asked of them and how that compares with the standard of care for their disorder.

7. There must be respect for both potential and enrolled participants. The participants must know the intended use of their information. This is particularly pertinent in the publication of case studies or pedigrees, where an individual might be unique and possibly identifiable, which could violate their confidentiality.

To ensure that these seven requirements are fully met, the proposal must be reviewed by a Committee on Ethics, referred to as the Institutional Review Board (IRB) in the United States.

When Is It Research?

In a few instances, it is not clear whether or not a clinical activity is research and requires administration of informed consent. If an investigator plans to publish any results of research on human subjects it must be reviewed by the IRB or Committee on Ethics. The ethics review may decide that the research is low risk, can receive an expedited review, and does not need a full review or it may be exempted from IRB review entirely. Examples of exempted research are anonymized records review. Expedited review may be used when questionnaires are used and individuals do not provide any personal identifiers when they return the questionnaire and their identity cannot be retrieved. However, no information gathered from a person may be published as part of a research study without their full knowledge that the process was part of a research investigation. Most biomedical journals now require that authors declare in the manuscript whether informed consent was administered to each of the participants and the protocol was approved by an IRB or ethics committee. Participants must be given the option to decline participation. If the activity meets any of the following criteria, it should be considered research:

1. The procedures being used or proposed are not the accepted standard of care for the disorder;

2. Data are being collected that are not required for the person's care;

3. The data will be published; or

4. The participant is being administered procedures for screening for a research study that they would not ordinarily receive as part of their regular care.

    If a case report involves procedures or testing that would not normally be applied for patient care purposes, IRB review and approval is needed. Also, a participant must give written permission for the use of their information for research publication purposes; this is particularly important in case reports where the individual might be identifiable.

What Are the Responsibilities of the IRB?

The IRB is responsible for ensuring that the study will have scientific validity, is of benefit to society, and does not pose undue risk of harm to participants. The questions addressed when an IRB reviews a research proposal are stipulated in 45 CFR 46 and are similar to the seven ethical principles listed above. These include:

1. Risks to participants are minimized;

2. Risks to participants are reasonable in relation to anticipated benefits;

3. Selection of participants is equitable;

4. Informed consent will be sought;

5. Informed consent will be documented;

6. The research plan makes adequate provision for monitoring the data collected to ensure the safety of subjects;

7. There are adequate provisions to protect the privacy of participants and to maintain the confidentiality of data;

8. There is an independent data safety and monitoring committee in treatment trials. This committee will examine the data in an unblinded fashion at regular intervals to determine if a trial should be stopped because of risks to participants or if a clear result has been obtained with a smaller number of participants than was originally planned.

Once the protocol is approved, the IRB is responsible for monitoring the conduct of the research through close communication with the PI and the research team. The IRB examines annual reports from the PI to determine if additional measures are required to ensure adequate protection of the research participants. The IRB must determine if: there are difficulties with progress of the study; any unexpected risks are being observed; and any changes are needed in the research procedures and/or the information contained in the consent. To fulfill these responsibilities, the IRB depends on the PI providing them with adequate feedback on the conduct of the research.

What Are the Responsibilities of the Principal Investigator to the IRB?

Although the principal investigator (PI) is responsible for developing the research protocol, once it is approved, the PI is responsible to the IRB to make certain that the approved research protocol is followed. The PI is responsible for guarding the rights, autonomy, and confidentiality of the participants in addition to preventing harm. The PI must ensure that the informed consent process is carefully executed (see below) and that the entire research team is adequately trained. Everyone involved must understand and follow the protocol. Before any changes are made in the conduct of the research these must be submitted as an amendment to the IRB for review.

Unexpected or serious adverse participant responses to the research procedures must be reported to the IRB as they occur (see below). It is of great importance to report all adverse events, whether expected or unexpected, related or unrelated, to the IRB. Serious and unexpected adverse events must be submitted in a written report within 7 to 15 days, depending on type, to the IRB.

Serious adverse events (SAE)s are those that result in death, are life threatening, cause hospitalization or a prolongation of hospitalization, disability, congenital anomaly, or require intervention to prevent impairment or damage. Further explanation for each category is provided in the FDA website at http://www.fda.gov/Safety/MedWatch/HowToReport/ucm053087.htm . Further considerations regarding serious adverse events are provided in a section below.

Expected adverse events, or those that are not serious, must be reported annually to the IRB. The staff and PI must also keep a running record of participants who withdraw from the research and the reason for their withdrawal. When reporting such information to the IRB, the PI should address whether the research procedures or the consent should be modified as a result.

What Are the Requirements for Informed Consent?

Informed consent, which provides the participant with a full understanding of the research and the ability to make an informed decision about participation or withdrawal, is essential for the involvement of human subjects in research. Regulations in 45 CFR 46 require that the informed consent document contain:

1. The purpose and need for the study and the procedures involved,

2. The possible risks based on the experience of prior participants in the research and on the research literature,

3. The possible benefits to participants that can be expected from the research,

4. The numbers of participants who have undergone the study and their experiences,

5. Disclosure of the appropriate alternative procedures or treatments that may be advantageous to the participant,

6. The parts of the protocol that are standard clinical practice and those that are the research components of the study,

7. The participant's reporting responsibilities to the research team,

8. The participant's rights to confidentiality and how their medical records, data, and research information will be safeguarded,

9. Assurance that information on their participation, diagnosis, and treatment will not be released without their written permission,

10. What compensation and/or treatment they will receive in return for participation in the research,

11. The participant's right to withdraw from the research at any time without their medical care being affected,

12. Whom to contact and contact information if they have questions about the research and in the event of a research-related injury,

13. Their right to information on any changes in risks as a result of others' participation in the research,

14. Accurate information regarding the time and inconvenience expected from participation in the research,

15. Assurance that they will be contacted if there will be any change in the use of their material by the investigators, and, if relevant,

16. Circumstances when participation might be terminated by an investigator without the person's consent.

WHAT IS GOOD CLINICAL PRACTICE BY A PI?

Good clinical practice in conducting a research study involves careful management of the protocol to ensure that the research team is closely following the research protocol and that any difficulties encountered are easily detected and addressed with timely and accurate reporting to the IRB when appropriate. Practices to ensure that these needs are met include the following:

1. Ensuring that each member of the research team has read and understands the research protocol,

2. Informing each member of the research team of their research responsibilities,

3. Training staff to conduct their responsibilities and to complete and follow checklists to make certain that all tests or procedures are administered as stated in the protocol,

4. Developing standard operating procedures to ensure that the procedures in the protocol are fully enacted,

5. Holding regular meetings with the research team to ensure that problems are identified early and discussed with the group,

6. Maintaining electronic databases on participants enrolled in the study, their completion of each phase in the research, outcomes, and follow-up,

7. Conducting regular quality assurance reviews at least annually of participant records to determine that consent forms are complete and each participant encounter, including telephone calls, are fully documented,

8. Maintaining a laboratory notebook of all events, including team meetings, decisions, and any difficulties encountered,

9. Ensuring that members of the research team document all events by stressing that if a procedure is not documented, it cannot be shown that it occurred.

The PI must be careful not to delegate important responsibilities, such as informed consent, without prior approval of the IRB.

WHAT IS SCIENTIFIC MISCONDUCT IN CLINICAL RESEARCH?

Examples of scientific misconduct in clinical research include: intentionally adding fabricated data (fabrication); intentionally altering records or intentionally deleting data or participants from the results (falsification); or using information not in the public domain, such as obtained from a manuscript or grant review without explicit permission of the other investigator (plagiarism). "Intent to treat" is of utmost importance; the research team must be careful not to exclude participants because they think that they would not respond well to the treatment being studied.

When misconduct occurs in a clinical research protocol or any research, all associated with the protocol may be under investigation and considered responsible, until it is resolved who was responsible (Office of Research Integrity, 2001, http://ori.hhs.gov/, p. 5). Persons to be investigated include: collaborators, technical staff, administrative support, data collection staff, statisticians, patient care staff, and the PI. Although the PI may have the primary responsibility for reporting to a panel during either an initial inquiry or an investigation of whether or not scientific misconduct has occurred, all members may be interviewed and all documents produced by members of the research team may be examined. To determine if data were fabricated, for example, the inquiry may need to examine the initial data recording, safeguards, and monitoring procedures followed by the PI and the research team to detect data entry errors, and whether or not the research procedures were followed by each member of the research team.

WHAT IS IRRESPONSIBLE RESEARCH CONDUCT?

Much of the irresponsible conduct in clinical research does not involve fabrication, falsification, or plagiarism, which are considered scientific misconduct. However, irresponsible conduct in clinical research is considered serious because it could result in harm or increased risk to research participants. Examples of irresponsible conduct include:

1. Violation of the protocol;

2. Incomplete records of subject participation or informed consent;

3. Not informing the IRB of participants' withdrawal;

4. Not protecting participants' confidentiality;

5. Not reporting unexpected adverse events or serious adverse events; or

6. Allowing conflicts of interest to bias the conduct of the research or interfere with the reporting of the research results.

Most of these examples are violations of the federal regulations contained in 45CFR 46, which apply to all federally funded research. Violations of federal regulations can result in censure of the PI or the staff, and/or suspension or termination of the research by the home institution, the IRB, or the Department of Health and Human Services Office for Human Research Protections. Some violations such as concealment of adverse events from the IRB could also be considered falsification or fabrication when done intentionally and are also examples of scientific misconduct.

WHAT ARE FREQUENT ERRORS IN THE CONDUCT OF CLINICAL RESEARCH?

Errors can occur in the conduct of research, which are unintended and are often due to poor management practices rather than intentional violations of federal regulations. The consequences can be just as serious, however, because they can bring harm to participants in the research and are considered non-compliant with Federal regulations (45 CFR 46). The following are examples of such errors and remedies to avoid such errors.

1. Including more participants in the study than were originally approved by the IRB. This can be avoided by maintaining an electronic database of all participants seen for the research and tracking their participation in each phase of the research. It is helpful to have one person responsible for maintaining the database and another member of the team conducting a regular review of the database. Limiting the numbers assigned to participants to the number approved for that group by the IRB will alert the investigator to when the maximum allowable participants have been accrued.

2. Including participants who do not meet the subject selection criteria. This can be avoided by using checklists during the screening process, and requiring that each entry be checked and initialed by the person doing the screening.

3. Failure to perform all of the tests required in the protocol. This can be avoided by requiring a staff review of participant's charts before allowing participants to enter the active phase of a study.

4. Not being aware of new information or research findings that would indicate an increase in risk to research participants. This can be avoided by using weekly or monthly automated bibliographic retrieval systems, such as Web of Science, Scopus, or PubMed, to alert investigators to new developments in a particular area of research.

5. Not being aware of recurrences of unexpected adverse events and not reporting these to the IRB. If such events are regularly recorded in a database,

they can be reviewed at regular intervals by the research team. Adverse events that are neither serious nor unexpected should be reported to the IRB annually with remedies proposed to avoid their recurrence.

6. Changes in the dosage or a treatment regimen without prior approval of the IRB can occur when new members of the research team are added. To prevent such errors, standard operating procedures (SOPs) should be written for guiding all members of the research team, and particularly for orientation of new staff when added to the project.

7. Not keeping records on participant encounters, procedures, and treatments. Good record keeping practices should be established and frequently reviewed by a staff member responsible for quality assurance. It is important to check that all participant records have the informed consent, procedure notes, test results, and case report forms, including telephone calls and follow-up notes.

Security of Participants' Records in Clinical Research

In clinical research, storage of research records can affect patient confidentiality. Servers containing patient records must meet HIPAA requirements. A recent concern is the role of portable media in storage of personal individual identifiers (pii) such as names, social security numbers, diagnoses, and so forth. In addition, institutions also are concerned about records of intellectual property (ip) that must not be available in the public domain. Many institutions now require that all portable media (laptops, hard drives, or flash drives) be encrypted and/or that "pii" or "ip" not be placed on any portable media.

MAINTENANCE OF RESEARCH RECORDS

Each member of the research team should maintain a laboratory notebook or record all actions into the ELN. As mentioned above, all entries should be written and dated in ink with no pages deleted and record decisions and discussions at team meetings, subjects admitted to the study, how procedures were conducted, data acquisition, coding, and statistical procedures. Because many database files are maintained on computers, the laboratory notebook should contain the names and location of these files for the study. The results of chart reviews for quality assurance and the occurrence and results of database reviews should be documented in a laboratory notebook. Many ELN programs can build in checks at each step to ensure that procedures are followed before the next step in the research can be initiated.

ADVERSE EVENTS

Adverse events are "any unfavorable and unintended diagnosis, symptom, sign (including an abnormal laboratory finding), syndrome or disease which either occurs during the study, having been absent at baseline, or, if present at baseline, appears to worsen" (Food and Drug Administration, 1995). These can include a participant getting a headache during testing or developing an upper respiratory infection within 2 to 3 days after participation. Adverse events may or may not be the result of an individual having participated in the research.

The PI is responsible for keeping the IRB fully informed on progress and any difficulties encountered during the conduct of the research. Adverse events must be reported annually. If recurrences of such events indicate that corrections are needed to avoid such events, the PI should propose new methods to the IRB to either reduce these and/or make changes in the consent form to alert future participants about the possibility of their occurrence. Participant withdrawal should be reported along with the reasons for withdrawal, which might indicate a need for changes in procedures, such as reducing the testing time.

To monitor for adverse events the PI should use nonleading questions of participants to record the outcome of their participation in the study. Asking, "Do you feel any different now, on completion of the study, from when you started the study?" and then recording the subject's response. Procedures and coding forms developed by the National Cancer Institute provide a routine method for classifying participants' adverse events (Cancer Therapy Evaluation Program, 1999) and are available at http://ctep.cancer.gov/protocoldevelop ment/electronic_applications/docs/ctcaev3.pdf.

SERIOUS ADVERSE EVENTS

Serious adverse events (SAE) fall into six categories and must be reported (FDA Form 3500A provides a good format for this) within strict timelines to the IRB, institutional authorities, and the FDA if part of an investigational drug or device trial. The six types of SAEs are those events that:

1. Result in death,

2. Are life threatening,

3. Require hospitalization or prolongation of hospitalization,

4. Cause persistent or significant disability/incapacity,

5. Result in congenital anomalies or birth defects, or

6. Are other conditions, which in the judgment of the investigators represent significant hazards.

Serious adverse events must be reported usually within 7 to 15 days depending on the type. Institutions must have procedures in place for prompt reporting when participants have been unexpectedly harmed or exposed to unanticipated risk (Title 45 Code of Federal Regulations Part 46, 1991).

When reporting on serious adverse events the PI should report:

1. Their judgment of the relationship of the event to the research,

2. Whether the event was expected or unexpected,

3. What actions were taken, and

4. The need to inform current or future participants on the protocol in the consent document or in writing about the serious adverse event.

Examples of SAEs include: aspiration of food followed by pneumonia requiring hospitalization, falls resulting in chronic injury, infections requiring hospitalization, nerve injury resulting in permanent or chronic paralysis, paresis, or paresthesia. Such instances must be reported if they occur while a participant is involved in a research protocol even if these are not the direct result of the research. The investigator should indicate when the event is part of the participant's underlying disease, if it has occurred previously, if there was a temporal relationship to the research, and if it is a reoccurrence of a previous or long-standing problem that predated the research. It also must be indicated whether or not any previous SAEs of the same type have occurred in the protocol.

WHO IS IN CHARGE OF THE RELEASE OF MEDICAL INFORMATION?

Because of the need to respect the rights of research participants and to prevent harm to participants, care should be taken not to release any information on an individual without their written permission. Because a person's insurance with third party payers might be affected by the knowledge of risk of illness, confidentiality of medical records has become an increased concern of participants in research. Only the participant can authorize the release of their medical information either to themselves or to others. Participants must be assured that their involvement in research will be confidential and diagnostic or treatment information will not be conveyed to others without their written permission. The written permission must be specific, stating who is to receive the information and what specific information is to be conveyed. Letters of referral or reports to a physician on a participant's care may only be sent with written permission of the participant who designates what material will be divulged. Unless there is a medical emergency and authorization is obtained from proper authorities, participants have the right to have information in their medical record withheld from others.

Contact with Family Members

Family members cannot be involved in discussions about the patient unless the patient has designated in writing that they are permitted to be involved in those discussions. When participants have a speech or hearing disorder and want investigators to communicate with a family member as their representative, written permission should be obtained before investigators discuss confidential medical information with a spouse or other family member.

Investigators must also take particular care not to correspond with patients or others through e-mail. This is not secure because copies are saved on mail servers and may be accessed illegally. Regular mail stamped "confidential" is the most secure way to convey information to participants. Faxes should be sent only when they are not being received in a public area and their receipt by the addressee can be ensured.

Special care is needed in genetic research, particularly because a person's family history may put them at increased risk of developing a debilitating illness. Release of such information, even when a person is unaffected, could do great harm to a participant if it prevents them from obtaining medical insurance or care. For this reason, care must be taken not to release information on participation in such research to others. Individuals should be asked whether or not they want their family members to know that they have participated in the study.

The development of pedigrees also must be done with great care. Members of the research team must not show family members pedigrees indicating who is affected and who is not. Such pedigrees divulge information on diagnostic status and will violate participants' confidentiality. Some members of a family may not want their diagnostic status divulged to others, even their immediate family members. When interviewing individuals, blank pedigrees must be used for this reason. Similarly, investigators and their staff must not compare one person's symptoms to those of another family member unless the participant volunteers the information.

WHAT ARE POTENTIAL CONFLICTS OF INTEREST IN CLINICAL RESEARCH?

Both financial and personal conflicts can interfere with the research process. When a pharmaceutical company has sponsored the research, the PI and staff should make certain beforehand that they have publication rights regardless of the outcome of the study. There can be significant financial incentives for both the pharmaceutical sponsor and the scientist to demonstrate benefit from a new drug. The same is true for research evaluating new medical devices. Future agreements with industry may depend on the outcome of an ongoing Phase 1 trial, which could bias the research results. When the PI has a patent pending, they may have a substantial bias that could interfere with the administration of treatment, the collection of the data, and the analysis.

Although financial conflicts have received the most attention, personal investment in the success of the research for reputation and career advancement are also strong incentives that can bias the research. Similarly, the PI may have a strong belief in the hypothesis being tested. Great care must be taken to include as many controls as possible to prevent bias from affecting the conduct of the study, data collection or analysis, and the interpretation of the results.

How Can a PI Prevent Problems?

Violations can occur in clinical research because the PI or members of the research team are not aware of the current rules and regulations. However, everyone involved in clinical research is responsible for ensuring that they are aware of such rules and regulations. The PI must ensure that staff members are conversant with current rules and regulations governing the conduct of clinical research. Annual refresher courses for PIs on the conduct of clinical research are now required.

Issues and questions often arise when members of the research team are uncertain about how to interpret the regulations or are not certain if regulations have changed. A quick e-mail to either the Chair of the IRB, the institution's Office of Human Subjects Research or Research Ethics Officer, or the DHHS Office of Human Research Protections can prevent problems. Persons in these offices are more likely to be conversant with the latest changes in regulations. Members of all these offices, particularly those at the home institution, would prefer to answer to questions and prevent potential violations.

Finally, documentation must be stressed to all members of the research staff. If an occurrence is not documented, there is no evidence that it took place. A regular quality assurance review will indicate how well the procedures in place are being followed.

ANIMAL RESEARCH

The use of animals for research is regulated by several sets of regulations and laws as follows:

1. The Animal Welfare Act (http://www.nal.usda.gov/awic/legislat/awa.htm) of the United States Department of Agriculture found in the Code of Federal Regulations Title 9, Chapter 1, Subchapter A, Parts 1 to 4. These regulations do not apply to birds, rat, or mice bred for use in research.

2. All investigators receiving funds for research support from the federal government, that is, the National Institutes of Health, the Food and Drug Administration, and the Centers for Disease Control and Prevention, must

be in compliance with the Public Health Service (PHS) Policy on Humane Care and Use of Laboratory Animals (http://www.nap.edu/readingroom/books/labrats).

3. The Office of Laboratory Animal Welfare in the Office of Extramural Research of the National Institutes of Health (http://grants.nih.gov/grants/olaw/olaw.htm) is the central reporting agency to which each Institutional Animal Care and Use Committee (IACUC) reports to regarding compliance with the PHS Policy on Humane Care and Use of Laboratory Animals.

4. The American Veterinary Medicine Association Guidelines on Euthanasia (http://www.avma.org/issues/animal_welfare/euthanasia.pdf).

Every institution that receives federal funds to support research involving laboratory animals must have an Institutional Animal Care and Use Committee (IACUC) that ensures compliance with each of the regulations listed above and reports to the Office of Laboratory Animal Welfare in the Office of Extramural Research of the National Institutes of Health. The IACUC is responsible for:

1. Reviewing animal use protocols and any significant changes in those protocols;

2. Evaluating institutional compliance with Public Health Service Policy, U.S. Department of Agriculture (Animal Welfare Regulations) and institutional policies;

3. Monitoring institutional animal care and use programs, and inspecting animal facilities on a regular basis;

4. Reviewing any concerns about animal care or use; and

5. Reporting noncompliance and suspensions to the Office of Laboratory Animal Welfare.

Investigators are responsible for complying with regulations and proposing research protocols to the IACUC, and once approved, following these approved protocols carefully to ensure that they are not deviating from the approved protocol.

Principles of Animal Care and Use

The major principles governing the use of animals in research are the 3Rs: reduction, refinement, and replacement.

■ *Reduction:* To use the least number of animals possible to answer a question, but to demonstrate that the investigation can answer the research question by having adequate numbers of animal to prevent erroneously failing to reject the null hypothesis

■ *Refinement:* To reduce to a species of least protection, to reduce procedures, and to minimize survival procedures that may cause pain or suffering

■ *Replacement:* Replace animals with computer models, and only use animals to verify the models.

There must be adequate rationale to justify the use of animals in research such as to determine how biology works, to develop disease models of pathogenesis of a disease, to test a model of pathophysiology of a disease, and to develop new treatments in an animal model of a disease.

A good relationship with the veterinarians is essential to using animals in research. It is advisable to meet with the head veterinarian before you start to develop plans to discuss your research, what species you will need, what housing and care support is required, the types of procedures, and in particular if you plan any survival surgery. The veterinarian's concerns are usually determining if you are knowledgeable about the procedures you are planning to conduct, what type of surgical training you have had, your knowledge of aseptic technique, what types of care is needed for the animals and how you will monitor them, and what experience you have with anesthesia. Postoperative care including monitoring schedules and intervention charts for possible care and problems that may develop and the persons responsible is essential. Euthanasia procedures must be humane.

Often, if you need training on a certain procedure, the veterinarians can help you with training; either they can train you or recommend an investigator on campus who is using that procedure and could train you.

Use of animals in research is dependent on controlling pain and suffering: every effort should be taken to avoid both. There are three categories: (a) no pain or suffering; (b) adequate alleviation of pain or suffering; and (c) no alleviation of pain or suffering. Obviously, categories (b) and (c) in particular are heavily scrutinized and must be very well justified.

ANIMAL STUDY PROTOCOL

Writing an animal research protocol emphasizes the numbers of animals to be used, the species to be used, and whether they are protected species such as nonhuman primates. Justification is needed to ensure that animals must be used, why the species is essential and adequate, and justification for the numbers of animals to be used. A literature review using several sources must demonstrate that the research is not duplicative. The procedures need to be detailed if surgery is involved and, most importantly, if survival surgery is included. Generally, the description should follow the animal from the start to finish demonstrating how pain will be controlled and euthanasia procedures. The details of postoperative monitoring and intervention criteria after survival surgery are needed. A separate section addresses anesthetic agents, dosages, and how they will be used.

Added documents are usually training forms for each investigator, intervention charts for animals after surgery, disposition of animals, use of radioactive materials, stem cells, and DNA recombinations.

Like clinical research protocols, care must be taken to review the approved protocol, avoid protocol violations, and if changes are needed to submit amendments and wait for approval before initiating them. The laboratory will be visited on a regular basis by the IACUC and they may question any member of the research team.

Finally, publication of the results is important; the use of animals is justified by adding to the knowledge base or impacting patient care.

7

Writing Research Proposals and Getting Funded

Writing research proposals requires training and practice, and is an acquired skill. Getting funded to do research depends on convincing the scientific reviewers and the program staff at an agency that the research is significant, novel, and well founded and will result in important new knowledge and/or improvements in patient care. Great care must be taken in presenting the proposed research; funding is not a matter or chance or luck, it totally depends on putting together a clear case for the importance of the research.

NATIONAL INSTITUTES OF HEALTH (NIH)

The NIH is the preferred federal government agency for external funding by many universities and research institutions. It is the largest federal agency to fund biomedical research. The premier grant awarded by the NIH is the R01 grant, an investigator initiated grant application. Many of the top R1 universities base the decision on tenure on whether the faculty member has been successful in obtaining an R01. The reason that the R01 is so highly prized is because it provides a national review of how well a person's research is recognized. An R01 award also provides income to the university or research institute that not only supports the individual's laboratory but also supports graduate students and provides indirect costs to the institution to support its research infrastructure and programs. Each institution has different policies for dividing up the indirect costs received, at some institutions some portion goes to the principal investigator's department. Another portion may go to the Dean to develop core research facilities to support several departments within a college.

The NIH receives its funds from Congress and the Director of the NIH must testify before Congress on recent achievements of the NIH in initiating and supporting research that addresses the overall mission of the NIH: to improve the health of the nation by conducting and supporting research (http://www.nih.gov/about/index.html#mission) (Figure 7-1).

The types of research and research training supported by the NIH are outlined further in Figure 7-2. In recent years, the emphasis of the NIH has enhanced support for research that addresses health needs. This is in part a result of pressure from Congress demanding results after doubling funding for the NIH in the 1990s. In 2006, Congress reauthorized NIH with P.L. 109-482, the National Institutes of Health Reform Act of 2006. This Act further emphasized the mission of NIH to focus on health and disease of the nation (http://www.nih.gov/about/reauthorization/index.htm).

The NIH is composed of over 27 institutes and centers (http://www.nih.gov/icd/index.html) supporting research in different research areas, often aligned with various diseases and/or medical specialties. The largest is the National Cancer Institute, which receives its own authorization and budget from Congress. Next in size is the National Heart Lung and Blood Institute, followed by several institutes such as the National Institute of Allergy and Infectious Diseases, National Institute of Diabetes and Digestive and Kidney Diseases, National Institute of Child Health and Human Development, National Institute of Neurological Disorders and Stroke, and the National Institute of Mental Health. Each of these institutes has its own mission and supports research in particular areas.

To meet its mission, the NIH:

1. Supports research through investigator-initiated grants,

2. Supports research training awards at the predoctoral, postdoctoral, and early career levels (only some institutes support predoctoral research training in high priority areas),

3. Awards research and development contracts initiated by research administration program staff on the advice of advisory groups when critical needs are identified as in need of support,

4. Provides research resources at many universities and medical schools, and

5. Conducts research on the NIH campus in Bethesda, Maryland, known as the Intramural Research Program.

The NIH also supports demonstration projects translating recent research advances into health delivery, supports research resources such as the National

Mission of the National Institutes of Health

NIH is the steward of medical and behavioral research for the Nation. Its mission is science in pursuit of fundamental knowledge about the nature and behavior of living systems and the application of that knowledge to extend healthy life and reduce the burdens of illness and disability.
The goals of the agency are as follows:
foster <u>fundamental creative discoveries</u>, innovative research strategies, and their applications as a basis to advance significantly the Nation's capacity to protect and improve health;

- •develop, maintain, and renew scientific human and physical resources that will assure the Nation's capability to prevent disease;
- •expand the knowledge base in medical and associated sciences in order to enhance the Nation's economic well-being and ensure a continued high return on the public investment in research; and
- •exemplify and promote the highest level of scientific integrity, public accountability, and social responsibility in the conduct of science.

FIGURE 7–1. Mission statement of the National Institutes of Health.

Programs Supported by the NIH

NIH provides leadership and direction to programs designed to improve the health of the Nation by conducting and supporting research:
- in the causes, diagnosis, prevention, and cure of human diseases;
- in the processes of human growth and development;
- in the biological effects of environmental contaminants;
- in the understanding of mental, addictive and physical disorders; and
- in directing programs for the collection, dissemination, and exchange of information in medicine and health, including the development and support of medical libraries and the training of medical librarians and other health information specialists.

FIGURE 7–2. Programs supported by the National Institutes of Health.

Library of Medicine, and is required to spend 2.5% of its funds on Small Business Innovation Research (SBIR) and 0.5% on Small Business Technology Transfer (SBTT) (http://grants.nih.gov/grants/Funding/sbirsttr_programs.htm).

Who's Who at the NIH

The organization and persons to contacts at the NIH can be confusing as there are several different types of administrators you will encounter during the grant application, review, and award process.

Program Directors

Of greatest importance are the "program staff" in each of the institutes at the NIH. Program Directors are Health Scientist Administrators (HSAs) who are responsible for monitoring programs and assisting scientists from around the country and internationally in a particular program area, such as a scientific or a disease area. They report to the Division of Extramural Research within an institute. Their responsibilities include being aware of major trends in an area of research, attending the peer review meetings where grants are reviewed, advising scientists who are applying in their area, and reviewing progress reports of grants assigned to them. They also attend the meetings of the National Advisory Council for their institute. An advisory council for each institute is comprised of external scientists and lay persons, each appointed for a four-year term by the Secretary of Health and Human Services. Advisory councils meet three times a year to make recommendations on funding, advise the director and staff of the institute on research needs, and may recommend a small number of grants that do not make the funding line for "special consideration" when the research addresses specific program needs of the institute. The program staff HSAs are the persons to contact after you receive a grant; they can provide advice on managing your grant, and when to apply for a competitive renewal. Program staff also develop program announcements and requests for applications when they identify areas of research needing attention and are given approval to emphasize a particular need by their institute director or their national advisory council.

If you are considering applying to an institute, you should first contact the member of the program staff who is responsible for research in your area. Usually the best approach is to send an e-mail with your Specific Aims page attached.

Training Program Director

If you are applying for a training award, there usually is an HSA program staff member in charge of training for each institute, sometimes in particular areas depending on the size of the program of an institute. Always contact the person in charge of training for that institute before you decide which type of award to apply for and whether or not an institute is interested in supporting training grants in your area.

Scientific Review Officers

Scientific Review Officers are scientists who serve as the Executive Secretaries of Review Panels or "study sections." Most are in charge of Scientific Review Groups (SRG) in the Center for Scientific Review (CSR), which is separate from the Institutes. Their responsibilities include identifying scientists to participate in grant reviews, making certain that the study section follows proper procedures, and editing reviews. The organization of the NIH can be confusing, but there are two sets of review groups, the majority are within the CSR (which is a separate part of the NIH). The reason for CSR being separate from the institutes is to maintain a two-stage review process: scientific review (totally focused on scientific merit) and program review, which is based on the mission of a funding source such as an institute. All grant applications go through the two stages of review unless they are excluded for particular reasons such as poor scientific merit, or difficulties with the protection of participants from research risks or animal care and use issues.

Institute Scientific Review Officers

There also are scientific review groups within the institutes for grants that are submitted in response to Institute Request for Applications such as Center grants (P50)s that cover a disease area or provide Core Support for research centers (P30)s. The Scientific Review Branch within an institute is separate from the program staff within the Division of Extramural Activities of an institute to keep the two stages of review (scientific and programmatic) separate. Scientific Review Officers within the Division of Extramural Activities in an institute may also be involved in the review of Small Business Innovation Research (SBIR) and Small Business Technology Transfer (STTR) programs.

FUNDING DECISIONS AT THE NIH

There are several levels of review of a grant proposal before a grant is funded with benefits and pitfalls at each level that must be considered when developing a research proposal. Most research proposals to the NIH are submitted through the Center for Scientific Review (CSR). On receipt, the CSR makes two assignments for a grant, first to the Scientific Review Group (SRG) also known as the "study section" based on the research content (Figure 7–3). This peer-review group of nongovernmental scientists will review the scientific merit of the proposed research, the budget justification and whether there are concerns about the use of human subjects for research or animal care and use issues. In addition, the use of children, minorities, and women in the research must be evaluated.

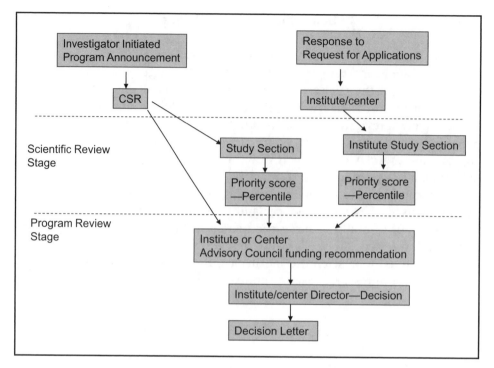

FIGURE 7–3. Grant Review Process at NIH.

At the same time, the CSR also assigns a proposal to an institute or center for funding consideration based on program relevance. Consideration for funding will occur after the proposal undergoes scientific peer-review by the study section or SRG. Sometimes, a grant proposal may have relevance to the mission of two institutes or centers, the CSR may communicate with each institute and one will take the lead assignment. It may be of advantage to have more than one institute available to fund the grant so the investigator should consider whether to include wording in their abstract and title that is relevant to the mission of more than one institute

The assignment to a study section for review and to an institute for funding consideration, are both based on the title and abstract of the grant proposal. Therefore, a close examination of the scientific areas of the different study sections is essential for determining which study section has expertise in the specialty area of the proposal and the PI. A careful review of the different study section rosters also is essential before writing your abstract to make certain that the appropriate study section is targeted (http://www.csr.nih .gov/Roster_proto/sectionI.asp#s). Each SRG/study section has a description of the areas of research that they cover and the current roster of standing members, although it is very likely that ad hoc members may be selected for a particular meeting to augment knowledge in a particular area not covered by standing members. Examining the mission statement and program areas of an institute is essential to make certain that your grant is assigned to the institute(s) that you think will be most interested in your work.

Some grant applications are submitted in response to specific announcements (either Program Announcements [PAs] or Requests for Applications [RFAs]) by an institute or center. In those cases the announcement, an RFA for a specific goal) or a PA (an announcement of a particular funding mechanism) is published in the NIH Guide to Grants and Contracts and may request that the application be submitted to the institute or center interested in supported research in that area rather than through CSR. Announcements expressing an interest in research using a particular support mechanism, usually PAs, may be submitted through CSR but should be identified as responding to a program announcement of a particular institute or center to influence programmatic assignment to the institute or center that has already expressed an interest in that area.

THE 2009 TO 2010 ENHANCING PEER REVIEW PROGRAM

Over a two-year period from 2009 to 2010, the Center for Scientific Review at NIH has revamped the peer-review system. This is aimed at reducing the administrative burden on research funding, identifying, and encouraging new and early stage investigators, streamlining the time from submission to award, and allowing NIH to fund the best science with the least amount of administrative burden. The new guidelines are available on the Web site (http://enhancing-peer-review.nih.gov) and in several new issuances:

- NOT-OD-09-023 which provides information on the implementation timeline for the new peer-review system,

- NOT-OD-09-024 on the new scoring procedures for the evaluation of research applications received for potential FY2010 funding, and

- NOT-OD-09-013 on revised new and early stage investigator policies.

The sections in this chapter on the scientific review process incorporate these new guidelines.

STUDY SECTION REVIEW

The study section or Scientific Review Group (SRG) usually contains between 12 and 24 standing members who are appointed for a 4-year term and meet three times a year. Some opt for a 6-year term with two meetings per year.

Most are midcareer scientists who have already been awarded R01s and are well regarded in their scientific areas. Generally, it is considered an honor to be appointed to a study section; however, the regular members work very hard to review a large number of proposals and take their responsibilities very seriously. Additional considerations enter into appointments such as the numbers of women and minorities on a study section and the geographic distribution of the reviewers. That is, care must be taken not to have too many members come from the same states.

The study section/SRG is convened by Scientific Review Officer (SRO) who may have a background in one of the areas covered by the study section/SRG. The SRO works closely with the Chair of the study section in assigning reviewers for each grant and identifying ad hoc reviewers when needed based on the content of the grant proposals assigned to the SRG for that cycle. Usually three reviewers are designated for a grant proposal and a reviewer may have many proposals (approximately 6 or so) to review in a cycle.

The first thing reviewers are asked to do before the meeting is to identify which grants have significant problems that will prevent them from being considered further, either because of poor scientific merit, ethical issues such as problems with the protection of human subjects for research, or animal care and use issues. Applications designated as not recommended for further consideration (NRFC) will not be referred to the Advisory Council for considerations for funding (Figure 7–4).

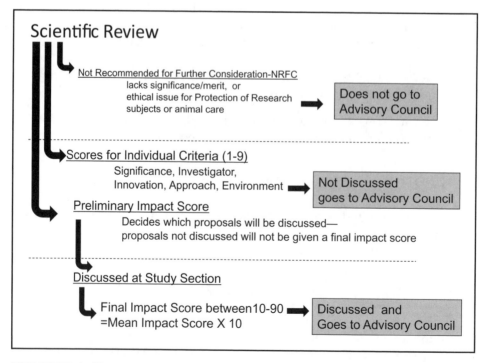

FIGURE 7–4. The possible outcomes of the NIH Research Grant Review Process.

Criterion Scores

Each application then will be evaluated by three reviewers who will be asked to provide criterion scores for five major aspects of the application: significance, investigator, innovation, approach, and environment. Each of these criteria will be rated on the same 9-point scale of 1 (high quality) to 9 (severe limitations). All applications will be scored in each of these categories. The three reviewers will also be asked to assign an overall preliminary impact score to determine whether or not an application should be discussed by the full study section. In general, only the top one-third is selected for discussion by the full study section. This selection is aimed at focusing on the merits of only those proposals that the preliminary reviewers consider as having potential for funding. This decision is based on the overall criterion scoring as well as the initial impact score (Figure 7–5).

Preliminary Impact Scores

The selection of the impact score is based on the table in Figure 7–5 where the ratio of the strength of the research proposal to the significance of the weaknesses determines the impact score. When there is a large range between the preliminary impact scores of reviewers, the SRO will encourage the three reviewers to read each other's reviews before deciding whether or not to recommend a grant for discussion by the full study section.

Those proposals that are "triaged" for not being discussed will receive 1 to 9 criterion scores on each of the five elements scored by the three

Guidance for Selecting an Impact Score

Impact	Score	Descriptor	Additional Guidance on Strengths/Weaknesses
High	1	Exceptional	Exceptionally strong with essentially no weaknesses
	2	Outstanding	Extremely strong with negligible weaknesses
	3	Excellent	Very strong with only some minor weaknesses
Medium	4	Very Good	Strong but with numerous minor weaknesses
	5	Good	Strong but with at least one moderate weakness
	6	Satisfactory	Some strengths but also some moderate weaknesses
Low	7	Fair	Some strengths but with at least one major weakness
	8	Marginal	A few strengths and a few major weaknesses
	9	Poor	Very few strengths and numerous major weaknesses

FIGURE 7–5. Guidance for selecting an impact score.

reviewers but no overall impact score. The PI will receive the reviews of the three reviewers and their criticisms that must be addressed in a resubmission.

The changes in the 2009 to 2010 Enhancing Peer Review Program have reduced the allowed number of resubmissions to one from the previously allowed two chances to resubmit, making it even more important to respond accurately to all criticisms on resubmission.

Final Impact Scores

Those grants in the top one-third are discussed at the study section meeting to concentrate the review on those within the funding range. At the meeting, the primary or first reviewer will describe the proposal for the full committee and give their review of each of the five criterion including the *significance* of the proposed research to the scientific field and patient care (if clinical) if it were successful, the *investigator's track record*, the *innovative* aspects of the research, the feasibility of the approaches proposed, that is, whether they are sound and can meet the specific aims proposed, and whether the research *environment* is supportive of doing the research. They will describe any concerns they have about the application as they pertain to each of the categories. Usually, the first reviewer is more descriptive of the project, giving some background, while the second and third reviewers state whether they are in agreement or disagree with the first reviewer and why. Each reviewer will propose a final impact score and then a scoring range is agreed on before each of the study section members votes their final score. The grant will be given an overall final impact score, which is the mean of the impact scores of each voting member of the study section. The mean score is then multiplied by 10.

Percentile Rankings

Percentile rankings are given to all grant applications reviewed by a study section over three consecutive meetings and are based on the impact scores. This then ranks a grant based on where the mean impact score falls in all the scored grants reviewed by a study section relative to other research proposals in the same field. The use of percentile ranks prevents one study section from rating all of their grants at a higher level, thus providing a greater chance of one field receiving more funding than others.

Often, one hears about the percentile score that an institute is able to fund to at a Council meeting. In times when budgets are small, sometimes as few as only the grants in the top 8th percentile rankings are funded, whereas when more funds are available, an institute may be able to fund to the 20th percentile. There also are differences between institutes in the percentile ranks they are able to fund. Some may have small grants and fewer commitments enabling them to provide a greater share of their dollars for new competing grants and such an institute can fund grants with higher percentile scores. The system is highly competitive and only a small percentage of grant applications receive funding, particularly in times of small federal budgets.

THE NATIONAL ADVISORY COUNCIL

After their review in CSR, grant applications with their percentile scores are then sent to the National Advisory Council of an institute for consideration for funding. The members of the National Advisory Council are appointed by the Secretary of the Department of Health and Human Services for a 4-year period. Some members are Senior Scientists in their field who have held grants for several years and served on study sections. Others are representatives from patient advocacy groups and lay organizations. Others have expertise in health care delivery, public health, or public health policy. The members of the National Advisory Council must approve all grants that will be funded by the Institute, although they do not make the final decision on funding, rather that is made by the Director of NIH, or the Institute Director as his or her representative. The final funding decision will depend on the amount of funds that are available for that council, usually approximately one-third of the funds that are left over after the institute has paid the previous commitments of grants previously funded for more than one year.

The funds available, therefore, depend on the funds allocated to the institute by Congress for that year minus the amount of funds required for commitments for that year for previously awarded grants and contracts. Also, the funds required to pay staff salaries (usually about 5% of the budget) and the costs for the intramural research program of the institute, which is usually around 10% of the total budget of an institute. Therefore, an institute usually will spend about 85% of the finds available on grants although only about 20 to 30% of that will be on new grants to be funded that year. There are three council meetings each year so that the money available for new grants is divided between the three council meetings. As a result, there will be a limited amount of funds available for new competing grants at each meeting of a national advisory council for an institute. Here, the percentile scores are used to rank each of the grants from highest to lowest. In most cases, the funds available are used starting from the highest percentile ranking (1st percentile) and go down to lower ranked grants in terms of percentile scores until the funds are spent. A very small amount of the funds may also be set aside for grants for "special consideration." This allows the staff and council members to give priority to areas of special need, such as research that has already been sought by the institute through requests for applications or program announcements.

THE DEVELOPMENT OF A GRANT APPLICATION

Given the highly competitive and rigorous system for awarding research grants, a great deal of care and work must go into the application. Starting early is essential.

Getting Started

Two Web sites are particularly helpful. First is the forms and instructions page of the Division of Extramural Research of the NIH (http://grants.nih.gov/grants/funding/phs398/phs398.html). This needs to be followed carefully, as the requirements for each section and budget are spelled out in detail. An excellent instruction guide on how to develop a research grant proposal and the process it goes through in review is available online (http://www.niaid.nih.gov/ncn/grants/cycle/default.htm) which takes an investigator through the entire process. Given the changes in the NIH grant application format, down from 25 pages to 12 pages, and the criterion areas to be judged, persons who were familiar with the old system will need to retool. A helpful book on the new system for both old and new NIH grant proposal writers is now available (Russell & Morrison, 2010).

Start early, particularly if this is your first research grant application to the NIH or NSF. You will need plenty of time to learn the process, write and rewrite your application, get input from others, and rewrite again and again. This is assuming that you have already gathered or published the necessary pilot data, had it analyzed, and that the results are adequate to support a research application. Although the extent of previous work in the area, pilot data, and previous publications to back up the application are less for training grants and exploratory grants such as R21s, all grants need some pilot data and R01s usually require publications as evidence that the procedures are known by the team. Usually 4 to 6 months in advance is advisable to begin writing, depending on teaching load and other responsibilities.

The Importance of Significance

This is an important component of the new NIH grant application; it is one of the five criterion scores. However, the definition of what is significant will depend on how well it matches the mission and priorities of the agency or foundation being applied to as well as what is of scientific significance for your field.

Given the importance of significance, which has increased greatly in recent years, the first goal in obtaining funding is finding a good match between your research aims and the mission of the agency or foundation—the first requirement to be considered. Although this chapter is aimed at submitting proposals to the National Institutes of Health, the guidelines presented here also apply to submitting proposals to the National Science Foundation and private foundations, except for important differences in mission, as will be explained later.

Although scientific merit also is of very high importance, significance is of equal importance, particularly when the target funding agency is disease-oriented such as a foundation interested in supporting research on a particular disease. Often, reviewers for a foundation are asked to score an application in two ways, one score for scientific merit and another for relevance to the mission of the foundation.

At the NIH, relevance to the mission as a whole of a particular institute or center is also significant. If your research is not aimed at a particular aspect of the mission of an institute, it may not be of interest to the program staff. Be certain to review each of the institutes or centers and find those that are interested in your area of research and contact the program staff early to get guidance on whether they might be interested, and also what types of support mechanisms are relevant to your application. For example, new investigators' applications (those who have not previously received funds from the NIH and are within 10 years of completing their terminal research degree or within 10 years of completing their residency) may be funded at a higher percentile from other R01 grant applications. Also, you might be qualified to apply for a training grant if you are at the predoctoral level, postdoctoral level, or may apply for a career development grant. Program staff at the institutes can be very helpful in guiding you on these aspects.

Start with the research proposal (part 2), leave the budget until the proposal is written, and the abstract usually comes last, after the entire proposal is written.

Specific Aims Page

The Specific Aims page is the first part of the project to start with and the most important. It is the introduction to the grant for the reviewer and must make it immediately evident why the research is being done, what the aims are (usually two or three are provided), the hypotheses to be tested within each of the aims, and the expected outcome of the research on the state of knowledge and/or patient care. Because the Specific Aims page will be sent to institute program directors as your first introduction, you should work on this with great care and get feedback from many persons before sending it to NIH program staff. It must make it clear to someone who does not have knowledge in your specific field that the proposed work will be important.

The format is now one page, starting with a paragraph on what the problem is and why it must be addressed. Then a short sentence or two is given for each of the specific aims, followed by the hypotheses to be tested for that aim with a sentence about its outcome.

Research Strategy (Significance, Innovation, and Approach)

This is the most important section and is now limited to 12 pages. It addresses three of the criterion areas; significance, innovation, and approach. It only leaves out the investigator (investigative team) and environment.

Significance must be written as an extension of the Specific Aims, providing an explanation of the need for the research and its import if successful. It must show the importance of the problem or how it is a critical barrier to progress in the field. The PI should explain how the current concepts, methods, technologies, treatments, services, or prevention that drive this field will be changed if the proposed aims are achieved.

Innovation must also be clearly spelled out; it must be apparent how this is new and not simply a replication of others' results. However, it should be shown how this also is the logical but a new first step to address the problem. Explain how the application challenges and seeks to shift current research or clinical practice paradigms. Describe any novel theoretical concepts, approaches or methodologies, instrumentation or intervention(s) to be developed or used, and any advantage over existing methodologies, instrumentation, or intervention(s). Explain any refinements, improvements, or new applications of theoretical concepts, approaches, or methodologies.

In the approach section, explain how the application challenges and seeks to shift current research or clinical practice paradigms. Emphasize any novel theoretical concepts, approaches or methodologies, instrumentation, or intervention(s) to be developed or used. The advantage over existing methodologies, instrumentation, or intervention should be made clear. Explain any refinements, improvements, or new applications of theoretical concepts, approaches or methodologies, instrumentation, or interventions.

Preliminary Studies/Progress Report

Preliminary studies must be included for new applications, particularly if published research by the PI or the investigative team cannot be cited. For a renewal application, a progress report must be included. References should be limited to those relevant to the project. The preliminary studies part of the application should prove to your reviewers that you are familiar with the techniques, have worked out the details, are skilled in the technological aspects of the work, and that results are assured. However, because of severe space constraints, previous publications are most useful. There is some truth to the belief that you must have already done a fair amount of the research to get it funded. Reviewers must be assured that you will be able to answer your questions and test your hypotheses.

Research Design and Methods

It is best to organize this section according to the Specific Aims and the hypotheses to be tested within each aim. Here is where you address alternative approaches and argue why you made the decisions to use the approaches you propose. Possible pitfalls should be addressed as at least one of your reviewers will likely have research experience in exactly the same area of research and as you have proposed. If you plan to use a consultant make certain they have read the proposal and have given you advice ahead of time that you are on the correct track. Their involvement should already be evidenced in the proposal. A letter of agreement will be required as an appendix.

For each Aim, there usually is an introductory paragraph giving justification and feasibility, then the hypothesis to be tested in Experiment 1. The research design, methods, and subjects, statistical methods, expected outcomes, and alternative strategies are the discussed. Then the same thing is done for Experiment 2, and so forth. At the end, a time-frame diagram can be presented and future directions may be discussed.

WRITING TIPS

Some writing tips are provided to make the application as readable as possible.

1. Do not use many acronyms; only those that are universal to science. A reader will become much less interested when they constantly have to look up abbreviations.

2. If possible, do not number references, as again this requires the reader to constantly refer to the bibliography.

3. Try not to be critical of others, they may be reviewing your proposal.

4. Never cite a reference unless you have carefully read the *entire* paper. The author of a paper may be one of your reviewers and will look on your proposal less favorably if you cite their work incorrectly.

5. Constantly refer back to the Specific Aims and the hypotheses throughout the document so that it is integrated.

6. Make certain you have shown how you will measure each of the outcome variables, and how they will be used to test each hypothesis.

7. Provide power analyses to demonstrate that your sample size is adequate to prevent Type II errors.

8. Make certain you have addressed possible pitfalls and alternate approaches to demonstrate you have thought through where problems might occur and how you can adapt to meet them adequately.

9. Format carefully to make the document easy to read. Insert diagrams and tables to clarify issues.

10. Follow the instructions carefully regarding font size and layout.

11. Provide clear justification for the budget items.

12. Don't assume that your reader is familiar with your particular specialty. Make certain scientists from other disciplines will understand the significance and why you have selected certain approaches.

SCHEDULE

First Month

Subscribe to NIH Guide for Grants and Contracts to receive announcements of new funding opportunities (http://grants.nih.gov/grants/guide/description .htm). Register with Commons list serve (http://era.nih.gov/about_era/get _connected.cfm). Speak to others who have been successful in the system for guidance and ask if they would be willing to review drafts for you and give you frank feedback. Well-funded senior investigators in your institution are best, in a related but not the same field. You should ask them if they would be willing to share with you a previous proposal that was funded, keeping in mind that the quality required for funding has become more and more rigorous—you will need to have as good if not an even better proposal.

Identify the target agencies for possible funding, reading mission statements for the institute or center. Search the NIH Guide for Grants and Contracts to identify program announcements, and request for applications that might be applicable to your research area. Draft your Specific Aims page with great care and, after many revisions, send it to some senior investigators for feedback. The Specific Aims page must state a significant problem that provides a logical background rationale for the aims of the study. Usually, there are two or three aims with specific hypotheses to be tested for each aim. The entire grant application will be framed around the specific aims and their hypotheses.

Contact a program administrator at each institute or center that you think might be appropriate to apply to for funding and send them your Specific Aims page by e-mail to determine if they are interested in your research. Follow-up with them by telephone if they indicate they are interested.

Second Month

Identify due dates for applying for the specific targets you are aiming at. Speak to persons in your institutional grants and contracts office to get any specific requirements they might have and make them familiar with your plans. Find out their requirements for submitting the grant through them. Discuss with them the registration process for electronic submission at (http://

www.grants.gov). The office of sponsored programs at large universities usually require that you send them the final application 2 to 3 weeks before the due date to make certain it is properly processed and approved by the university authorities in time for submission.

Download all the applicable forms, learn the submission process, and register in eRACommons (https://commons.era.nih.gov/commons/index.isp ?menu_itemPath=Home). The NIH now uses a completely electronic submission process that needs to be approached well in advance—not at the last minute. See SF424 Research and Related (R&R) forms and the SF424 (R&R) Application Guide (http://grants.nih.gov/grants/funding/424/index.htm). Start writing by first revising your specific aims. Keep in mind that the specific aims provide the hypotheses, the rationale, and the significance of the research. The entire grant will carry those themes throughout so that you can demonstrate that you will be able to provide a clear test of the hypotheses.

The hypotheses must have importance for the field at large. You are requesting taxpayer funds to support your research; therefore, your research must be of importance to the society at large. Descriptive research does not rank well as it cannot be assured that significant new knowledge will be gained. By having hypotheses, it is assured that answers will be obtained and these should provide important new information that will move the field forward.

While writing you should keep in mind that you must be in the top 10% to be funded; some institutes will only be able to fund the top 8th percentile of scored applications. Currently, well over 60% (the majority) of applications are "triaged," that is they are not discussed at the meeting of the study section and the PI will receive the reviews of the two or three reviewers who were assigned the grant to review. In fact in recent years, the goal is to triage close to 70% to allow the reviewers to discuss in more depth only those applications that have some possibility of being funded.

With the new review system, feedback on the review is provided much earlier, allowing investigators the opportunity to revise and resubmit before the next submission date.

Third Month—Completing the First Draft

By the end of the third month you should have a well-written draft of the grant proposal that is almost complete. This will be used to get others' input and agreement to participate if you have collaborators or consultants. Always use a confidential background on all text that you send to others and send it in the ".pdf" format to discourage others from intentionally or unintentionally copying your materials. Give people at least two weeks, usually three, but remind them if they have agreed to give you feedback. Often, asking them to give you a telephone call can reduce the need for them to waste time writing out their feedback; also, you will get more straightforward feedback on the phone or in person.

Fourth and Fifth Months

You will be rewriting based on comments from reviewers. Ask persons in your field who have served on a study section (but not ask those currently on study sections or they will have to exclude themselves from review). Also ask senior scientists at your institution who might not be very familiar with your specific discipline.

Often, let it sit for 2 weeks before going back to it; often you can see where the problems lie after you take a break. Keep reviewing the literature to make certain you have not missed something.

Start meeting with your office of sponsored programs after the fourth month on programming a budget sheet in Excel so that when changes are made you do not have to reconfigure the budget each time, it will automatically do that for you. Make certain you get it to the office of sponsored programs early so that there is plenty of time for review, approvals, and input. Remember there are likely many other scientists on campus trying to meet the same deadline and that all have to go through the same office of sponsored programs. You will get less attention and assistance if you wait to the last minute.

RESUBMISSIONS

Most research proposals do not receive funding on the first review; a large number need to be resubmitted to be funded. Be certain that you carefully address each of the initial criticisms as the reviewers the second time around will have your previous review or "pink sheet" and you must be responsive to all the criticisms in the previous review. Always resubmit, if you do not you will certainly not be funded. You can only be funded if you resubmit.

SPECIFIC TYPES OF GRANTS

The majority of grant application are R01 grant applications, which are the gold standard of the grant awarding system. Some other types may apply.

Academic Research Enhancement Award (AREA R15)

These are aimed at primarily undergraduate universities to enhance the research involvement of undergraduate students. A university can be designated as an AREA institution if it has not been a major recipient of NIH support. Applicants may request up to $300,000 direct costs plus applicable Facilities & Administrative/indirect costs for the entire project period of up to three (3) years. The total amount awarded and the number of awards will depend on the mechanism numbers, quality, duration, and costs of the applications received (http://grants1.nih.gov/grants/guide/pa-files/PA-06-042.html). Be certain to speak with program staff for further direction and on whether the guidelines differ for this program by institute.

R21 Exploratory/Developmental Grant

This type of grant is not common to all of the institutes and in fact, many NIH program staff now consider this mechanism to have been a failure as it has not produced many successful R01 grants. This mechanism is intended to encourage exploratory and developmental research projects by providing support for the early and conceptual stages of these projects. These studies may involve considerable risk leading to a breakthrough in a particular area, or the development of novel techniques, agents, methodologies, models, or applications that could have a major impact on a field of biomedical, behavioral, or clinical research (for example, http://www.nidcd.nih.gov/funding/types/researchgrants.asp#R15).

NIH Small Research Grant Program (Parent R03)

This is a small grant program again only used by some institutes (http://grants.nih.gov/grants/guide/pa-files/PA-09-163.html). Applications may be submitted for up to four modules of $25,000 each ($100,000 total direct costs per year), for up to three years of support. No renewals are allowed.

TRAINING FELLOWSHIPS AVAILABLE

(See http://grants.nih.gov/training). The F30 is for predoctoral candidates seeking the combined degrees of MD/PhD. There are a series of predoctoral fellowships, F31, particularly aimed at minority candidates. The F32 is aimed at support for postdoctoral research training. The F33 is for senior fellows who want to make changes in the direction of their research career by learning new techniques and are applied for directly. The T32 is an institutional research training grant given to high-quality research training programs. Potential candidates at the predoctoral and postdoctoral levels can search for these on NIH RePORTER to see what is available in their area of interest.

Career Development Grants

At last count there were at least 14 different types of K awards that are aimed at candidates who are new investigators, after postdoctoral study and need salary support to allow them to further develop their research program to prepare to apply for an R01 grant. Often the institution has to show that the candidate is tenure track and that they have a long-term commitment to the candidate. Given the complexity of the K award system there now is a questionnaire available online to allow you to answer questions that direct you to the correct type of award to apply for. Many are only offered by some institutes. Some are for persons in the basic sciences (http://grants.nih.gov/training/kawardresearch.htm), whereas others are for candidates in health professional doctorates (http://grants.nih.gov/training/kawardhp.htm). Most of these awards provide for 3 to 5 years of salary support and some laboratory support to enable the candidates to be mentored as they progress towards submitting and receiving their own R01 funding.

Overall, the aim is to have mechanisms available to allow young scientists to progress through stages of less and less mentorship and training until they are ready to establish their own laboratory with full grant funding. The first step in applying for career development grants is to develop a short one-page synopsis of your career stage, the type of training you need, the specific aims, and the type of K grant you are considering applying for. This should be sent to a training director at an institute or a program staff to get their guidance on which mechanisms you would be eligible for and which mechanisms the institute is emphasizing for person with your scientific background and training.

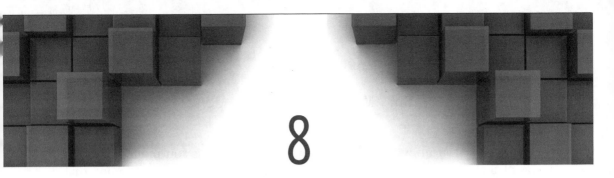

8

Career Paths Outside Academia or Away From the Bench

*D*uring their graduate work, scientists-in-training are exposed largely, and sometimes exclusively, to the academic career. PhD mentors hold faculty positions and spend all or most of their time in academic settings (although some participate in research in nonacademic settings such as industry). Not surprisingly, many newly minted PhDs restrict their job searches to the world of colleges and universities and begin to think of their career goals solely in terms of academic traditions (teaching, tenure, faculty committees, and so on). But PhD graduates have skills and abilities that apply to a variety of nonacademic workplaces and a variety of job responsibilities. Considering these nonacademic opportunities is appropriate for a number of reasons such as: an oversupply of PhDs for the available positions in some academic specialties, finding a position that is ideally suited to individual interests and abilities, developing a career plan that involves a combination of employment settings and responsibilities, and focusing on research without having other obligations such as those typical of academia.

This chapter considers scientific careers in a number of different work settings and explores careers that are removed from the laboratory bench. The employment opportunities considered here by no means exhaust the possibilities. Scientists are suited to many different jobs, and there is reason to believe that the employment spectrum will expand as science continues to grow in its influence on virtually all aspects of society. In all likelihood, the spectrum of scientific careers will continue to expand, with some future jobs yet to be defined.

SOFT MONEY VERSUS HARD MONEY

What does it mean when someone says, "My position is soft money but I am applying for another position with hard money?" Soft money is funding that depends solely on grants and contracts, without guarantee of salary support from other sources if the grant or contract expires. This kind of funding is "one-time" only and generally comes from federal or private sources. Hard money is funding secured by a long-term contract or agreement with an institution and does not depend on extramural grants or contracts. University faculty positions are a good example of hard money, because the institution usually honors its salary commitment even if extramural sources of support are not continuous. The primary difference between hard money and soft money is that the former carries the assurance of continuous support for salary (but not necessarily support of a research lab), whereas the latter involves short-term salary commitments. Soft money does not always mean that a position will come to an end in the near term, but that possibility must be recognized. Hard money does not mean a lifetime guarantee of employment and it certainly is not a sinecure.

Scientists who are supported entirely by soft money receive their salary support from grants and contracts that usually are administered by government or private organizations. Because these scientists receive little or no salary support from their immediate employer, they are not obligated to substantial work responsibilities outside the scope of work defined in their grants and contracts. Scientists who are fully supported by soft money can devote nearly all of their time and effort to the grant or contract. The advantage of this focused effort is offset by the uncertainty of funding. Consider the example of a scientist employed by a university in a nonfaculty rank (e.g., a scientist position). So long as the scientist is successful in obtaining extramural funding, he or she can conduct research that is supported by the funding agency. But if the funding ceases, the university has no obligation for salary support and the scientist may have to look for another position or seek alternative sources of support that would ensure continuation of the scientist position.

Scientists on soft money may feel that they are on a treadmill of proposal writing to ensure their salaries and the continuity of their research labs. Writing grants can seem like a vicious cycle, given that in the current climate, only rarely is a research application funded on its first submission. When a proposal is not funded, the scientist has to revise the application and wait for another cycle of submission and review, a process that takes 9 to 12 months. The new NIH review process will shorten the cycle, but it is inevitable that delays will be experienced. Furthermore, government effort-reporting requirements prohibit researchers from using grant funds for grant writing or any other activity not directly related to the research outlined in the grant. Some scientists thrive on the competitive nature of soft-money support, but others find it to be an unrelenting and anxiety-producing experience that has uncertain rewards.

Soft-money positions in universities, research institutions, and some other enterprises may have distinct career tracks. For example, most universities have tracks designated by terms such as "scientist tracks" that are different from faculty or professorial tracks. Scientist tracks typically do not lead to tenure, although some individuals initially hired on such a track may be placed into a tenure-track position. The scientist track is geared to the needs of research, which is appealing to many who hold these positions. On the other hand, universities are oriented strongly around faculty positions, and it is the faculty who serve on the majority of committees and often have the most say in fiscal and policy matters. At least a few individuals on nonfaculty appointments chafe under the hierarchical pattern of academic decision making.

The soft versus hard money issue can take different forms during a career. A tenure-track appointment in academia is hard money in the sense that job security is ensured once tenure is granted. But until a positive tenure decision is made, the position does not carry a guarantee of career-long employment. Therefore, the salary commitment is "hard" only for the length of the initial appointment. As another example, consider a tenured university scientist who assumes a position as laboratory director that depends on the funding of a large research grant. The director position could be terminated if funding is terminated, and the individual may then return to a professorial position.

FEDERAL EMPLOYMENT

The federal government employs a large number of scientists and engineers (just over 200,000 in 2005, with about 123,000 of this number being scientists). The agencies employing the greatest number of individuals in these categories are, in descending order, the Department of Defense, Department of Agriculture, Department of the Interior, Department of Health and Human Services, Department of Commerce, National Aeronautics and Space Administration, Environmental Protection Agency, and Department of Veterans Affairs (data from National Science Foundation, Infobrief, 2009, http://www.nsf.gov/statistics/infbrief/nsf09316/nsf09316.pdf).

Federal jobs offer security and relatively good compensation. There are several different pay systems, but eight are predominant. Approximately half of the federal workforce is under the General Schedule (GS) pay scale, 20% are paid under the Postal Service Rates, and about 10% are paid under the Prevailing Rate Schedule (WG) Wage Grade Classification. Other pay systems include the Executive Schedule, Foreign Service, Nonappropriated Fund Instrumentalities pay scales, and Veterans Health Administration. GS employees are considered white collar workers under the federal classification system. Each

GS grade has 10 pay steps, with steps earned based on time in service and work performance. Recently, most federal agencies have implemented "pay for performance" programs. Employees are placed in core compensation pay bands, and compensation is determined by performance rather than by automatic increases in General Schedule steps.

The Book of U.S. Government Jobs (Damp, 2008) is a highly informative introduction to the federal hiring process. In addition, it includes government and private sector Web sites, electronic bulletin boards, self-service job information centers, telephone job hotlines, and other resources pertaining to searches for federal employment. It contains advice and materials on resume development and job applications. As of September 2006, the federal government's civilian workforce numbered about 2.7 million, and about half of them are currently eligible for either early or regular retirement. Accordingly, the prospects for future government hiring are very strong.

Although over 80% of the budget of the National Institutes of Health is spent on grants throughout the United States and in some foreign countries, the NIH also has laboratories and a research hospital on the campus where scientists work in the Intramural Research Program largely on the campus in Bethesda. Most institutes have intramural programs where they recruit investigators to run research programs/laboratories in their area of expertise. The principal investigators usually have a small group of scientists who, along with postdoctoral fellows, work in a research area. The principal investigators become tenured after a rigorous tenure track review system and are subsequently reviewed by external scientists every 4 years to assess their scientific contributions and plans. Their resources are dependent on how they do in the review system and the decisions are made by scientific directors of the intramural program of the institute. Staff scientists work under principal investigators usually on 5- to 7-year renewable contracts. Each principal investigator will have an average of 4 or 5 postdoctoral fellows who train with them for 2 to 3 years before going on to tenure track positions in academia. Position openings at the NIH are advertised online and in scientific journals, and scientific job openings can be searched at USAJOBS for NIH and the Veterans Administration (http://jobsearch.usajobs.gov/search.aspx?brd=3876&vw=b&FedEmp=).

The Department of Veterans Affairs employs scientists in its Biomedical Laboratory Research and Development Service (BLR&D) and Clinical Science Research and Development Service (CSR&D). Principal investigators in these intramural programs are expected to conduct scientific research, but also to participate in committees, direct core facilities, teach, mentor, supervise shared resources, and perform other kinds of activities related to the research mission. The career track for nonclinician scientists at BLR&D and CSR&D are: (a) research scientist, (b) research career scientist, and (c) senior research career scientist. The first of these is conferred based on funding of a VA Merit Review Award Program (MERIT). The latter two designations are conferred by appointment in recognition of outstanding achievements and contributions to VA research. Salary support is provided for the term of the award and is indefinitely renewable.

MEDICAL SCHOOLS

Research in medical schools is conducted mostly by PhDs and MD-PhDs. Although the latter have clinical training, they may not have or elect not to have clinical responsibilities. As a rule, scientists who work in medical schools have a reduced teaching load compared to those who work in nonmedical academic departments. Frequently, the teaching expectation in medical schools is restricted to a few lectures given to medical students or residents. In contrast, the teaching load in a nonmedical department ordinarily is two courses per academic term in a research-intensive university and as much as four courses per term in colleges or universities that do not place such an emphasis on research. The courses may include large-enrollment undergraduate courses, with or without a laboratory section. When other responsibilities, such as committee service, student advising, and mentoring, are added to the mix, the demands on a faculty member's time can be challenging.

Scientists who are interested in medical school appointments should be aware of trends in the nature of these appointments. First, although the percentage of full-time, nontenure track basic faculty has been increasing (8% increase from 1980 to 2000), the percentage of basic science faculty on nontenure track appointments is increasing relative to the percentage with tenure-track appointments. This pattern is rooted in several factors: (1) a pattern in some schools of appointing new faculty to nontenure-eligible faculty tracks such as research scientist positions, (2) hiring new faculty members on 100% soft money, and (3) reappointing faculty on nontenure tracks to tenure tracks as they establish their success.

A second major trend is a change in the financial guarantee attached to tenure. A guarantee of total institutional salary for basic scientists is being reduced, largely as a hedge against budget uncertainties. For example, a university or research institution may guarantee only half of a scientist's salary on the assumption that the remainder will be covered by research grants or contracts. Such an arrangement is further incentive for a scientist to maintain extramural funding.

The third trend is toward increased latitude in pretenure policies, including lengthened probationary periods, changes in up-or-out provisions, and allowing faculty to switch between tenure and nontenure tracks. This flexibility can offer advantages to scientists but it also comes with some risks. For example, one potential disadvantage is that lengthened probationary periods extend career uncertainty because of a delayed tenure decision.

INDUSTRY AND PHARMA

Employment growth for scientists in this sector is anticipated on the promise of advances in medical devices, biologics and biopharmaceuticals, food, renewable energy, and renewable materials, to mention but a few. A valuable source of information is on careers in biotechnology is the Biotech Work Portal (http://www.biospace.com/bwp_careers.aspx).

Scientists employed in industry or pharmaceutical companies have less autonomy than researchers who work in academic settings. The research agenda in private industry is strongly influenced by market considerations so that scientists may have to explain and defend their work in terms of a business plan that has a profit motive. There also will be an emphasis on project deadlines geared to schedules of product development and release. Although scientists may have some self-determination with regard to their projects, the latitude is greatly reduced relative to scientists in academia.

According to one set of recent data (http://www.diversityworking.com), the employment of medical scientists breaks down as follows: 30% in scientific research and development services firms, 24% in government, 14% in pharmaceutical and medicine manufacturing, and 13% in private hospitals. The majority of the remainder were employed by private educational and ambulatory health care services. Only about 1,000 were self-employed.

Scientists sometimes work in "business development," a term that can have very different meanings depending on the size and nature of a company. In small companies, business development may be nearly equivalent to a sales position, but in large companies, business development can refer to strategic and market planning, business development, and licensing. Business-development positions tend to be more specialized in large companies and may involve searches for new products, adapting products to new markets, or developing strategic partnerships. Business experience may not be absolutely necessary for these positions, but applicants may increase the likelihood of being hired if they can demonstrate relevant career experience or training (which can range from a few online courses to a Masters of Business Administration).

Scientists who decide to apply for positions in industry or pharma should recognize the cultural differences between academia and the private sector. Some of the accomplishments that curry favor in academia will mean little or nothing in the business world. This is not to say that academic experience is irrelevant but rather that the experience should be cast in terms that are relevant to profit-making enterprises. In applying for positions outside of academia, scientists should take a hard look at their CVs and ask how the information can be packaged to be more appealing to private industry. A first step is to identify skills that are useful, and even critical, in the private sector. One of these is oral and written communication. To demonstrate this kind of skill, it rarely is sufficient to provide a reprint of a highly technical article. The point might be made more powerfully by showing an example of a "plain language" article that succinctly and clearly describes a scientific phenomenon. The point is that communication that matters is not only between individuals with shared technical expertise but between individuals with different and complementary expertise. Another example of a skill that transfers from academia to industry is the management of projects and resources. It is well to remember that experience in problem-solving, analytical thinking, staff supervision and training, and brainstorming is relevant to virtually all employment settings. Another personal trait to be emphasized is self-initiative, to show that you can apply your skills and intelligence to forge new projects and point the way to new directions. It is better if you can show how you persuaded others of the value of these plans. For this reason, the resume should be written so as to point out particular accomplishments, especially the development of innovative approaches or materials, successful collaboration in a complex undertaking, or participation in a long-range development project.

Employment in the private sector also can mean a different pattern of working compared to that in academia. One of the advantages of an academic life is the ability to select the work focus for a particular period of time. In addition, academics usually move from one task to another on a weekly or even daily basis. For example, a faculty member may spend a day as follows: writing a paper in the early morning, meeting with a graduate student to discuss the student's research project, giving a lecture to a large undergraduate class, attending a brown-bag research seminar, meeting with lab personnel to review recent progress, teaching a graduate-level class, and finally reviewing a set of grant proposals. Switching between tasks can be difficult at times, but such variation also tends to prevent boredom with any particular task. In contrast, a scientist employed in the private sector may spend all or most of the day on a single task, such as working at a computer to complete a complex data analysis, or writing a technical report on a project in progress. Furthermore, the daily activities may be determined by a supervisor or company executive, who expects that the scientist will apply him- or herself to the task at hand, with little or no interruption. This top-down management style is typical of corporations but not academia. Not surprisingly, some scientists who have an academic background and move to the corporate world may find it disconcerting at first to find that someone else tells them what to work on and when to get it done. Of course, the very successful scientist eventually may be the one who gives the orders to others in the corporation.

RESEARCH ADMINISTRATION

Universities, research labs, government, and businesses that have a substantial involvement in research rely on administrators with a scientific background to oversee and direct research activities. These administrative positions differ somewhat in job description across settings but they usually emphasize administrative and interpersonal skills in addition to scientific knowledge. Because these positions carry budgetary authority over colleges, departments, or other administrative units, they require financial skills. In addition, these positions entail the ability to see the bigger picture, envision the future, and grasp complex connections across disciplines. There can be a considerable tension between fiscal responsibility and risk-taking. Naturally, a high-level administrative position is suited to individuals with considerable experience, so this kind of job is not entry level. Anyone interested in research administration can begin to learn about the responsibilities of such a position by volunteering for committee service, applying for full- or part-time positions that will provide experience, or by participating in workshops and seminars that focus on relevant job skills.

Many midcareer scientists choose to move into Health Science Administrator (HAS) positions at the National Institutes of Health in the Extramural Programs. These can be excellent new career opportunities for those who no longer want to be at the bench but want to work in having a leadership role in their scientific discipline and beyond. Some become program officers responsible for developing and shaping the future directions of a scientific area. Responsibilities are to identify new opportunities for developing new knowledge or improving the prevention, diagnosis, or treatment of disease. Program officers at the NIH evaluate progress in areas of science and can convene panels of scientists to emphasize new directions. Program officers are also advisory to scientists in the field helping them find which mechanisms are best suited to their particular situation in applying for research support. They also read the progress reports from the grants in their specialty area and report on the state of the field to institute directors. They are responsible for program announcements and request for applications to increase scientific interest in new areas that can address program needs.

Other HSA positions are in the Center for Scientific Review or in Scientific Review Branch of an institute. Here a scientist uses his or her knowledge in an area to select reviewers for applications and shapes the feedback from a review for the applicants so that they can follow the review directions.

Other scientists work in government in the Department of Health and Human Services, either in the Office of Research Integrity reviewing investigations of misconduct or in the Office for the Protection for Human Research Protections reviewing cases of noncompliance with regulations concerning the use of humans in research. As scientists progress in these positions they can be promoted into policymaking positions that can have a major impact on research policies that they could have never achieved being a bench scientist.

ALTERNATIVE CAREERS

Careers in this category are those that have not been traditional for scientists. The term "alternative careers" is not really apt because it connotes something unusual or exceptional. In fact, these careers are becoming increasingly common. It also is not particularly useful to call these careers "nontraditional" because that term is a negative definition that assumes a common understanding of what is traditional. Perhaps it is best to think of the careers in question as "new horizon careers" because they are part of what is likely to be an ever-expanding horizon of career possibilities that are defined by the important role of science and by the ingenuity of scientists.

Scientists are experts in a particular discipline, but they also acquire a variety of skills that can be useful in many different careers. The skills include problem solving, technical writing, review and evaluation of scientific projects, interpretation of scientific results for specialty and general audiences, collaborative planning, and consulting on research. Careers that do not involve bench science include public policy specialist, technical writer, technical service support, biotechnology sales representative, patent attorney, patent examiner, technology transfer officer, field application specialist, clinical trial design implementation and monitoring, quality assurance specialist, science journalist, science textbook editor, and consultant to nonprofit organizations. These are only a sampling of possible positions and are not intended to be an exhaustive list of alternative careers. Many of these careers draw heavily on scientific expertise, including knowledge of specialized instruments and laboratory procedures. As science has a continuing growing impact on society, there will be an increased demand for bench scientists and other scientifically trained individuals who can evaluate and translate scientific discoveries. PhDs in science should take a lesson from graduates from law school who use their legal training to good advantage in a variety of work settings. After all, the PhD reflects highly developed reasoning and interpretive skills, along with laboratory expertise and communication abilities.

EXPLORING THE POSSIBILITIES

Trying out a career before making a definite commitment is a possibility in some fields. An internship, a part-time appointment, or job-shadowing is a way to learn about a career alternative. In certain areas, postdoctoral fellowships and other kinds of support are available to enable scientists to explore alternative careers. Some possibilities are the following:

AAAS Science and Technology Policy Fellowships:
http://fellowships.aaas.org/

AMS-AAAS Mass Media Fellowship:
http://www.ams.org/government/massmediaann.html
(This 10-week summer fellowship is designed to give graduate students in mathematics an opportunity to intern at mass media organizations)

Knauss Fellowship: http://www.seagrant.noaa.gov/knauss/index.html
(This is a NOAA fellowship for ocean, coastal, and Great Lakes policy)

NSF Science, Technology, and Society postdoctoral fellowship: http://www.nsf.gov/funding/pgm_summ.jsp?pims_id=5324&org =SES&from=fund

FINDING A JOB

A piece of advice that occurs repeatedly on Web sites, articles, and Q&A forums is that it is not enough to look at want ads to find a suitable job. This approach often is fruitless and frustrating. Networking is recommended as the best way to learn about possible openings, to discover new developments related to employment, to announce your availability, and to advise others of your particular skills and experience. Networking is not simply schmoozing or glad-handing at receptions and interviews. Rather, networking is a skill to be cultivated. It draws on research (e.g., to discover the product line of a company), making contacts, diligent preparation to communicate one's expertise and interests, and acute listening and looking to pick up on nuances that might lead to deeper discussions of possible employment.

Especially if a job search extends across various academic and nonacademic sectors, it can be helpful to prepare alternative versions of a resume, ranging from a highly condensed single page with bulleted descriptions to the traditional curriculum vitae that covers all the bases. Ask others to review your resume or CV and give their frank assessment of whether it is successful and appropriate for different kinds of careers. In applying for jobs in the private sector, one approach is to emphasize knowledge, skills, and abilities (KSA), as this kind of description enables prospective employers to grasp immediately the qualifications most suited to their needs.

SETTING CAREER GOALS

As discussed in Chapter 1, it is important to set realistic goals and define steps to reach them. A resume or CV is a useful tool to summarize career accomplishments for oneself as well as for employers and supervisors. Updating these documents is one way to keep a fresh perspective on career development, including skills acquired, responsibilities discharged, and projects completed. Especially for those who may change positions or combine careers (e.g., a part-time position in academia and another part-time position in industry), it is good to maintain both a resume targeted for the private sector and a CV directed to academic circles.

Setting career goals establishes a pattern of decision-making that operates both in the short and long term. For instance, an invitation to take on a new responsibility may be a valuable step toward a long-range career objective. Goals are not written in stone. They can be revised and often are. Changing a goal should not be viewed as an admission of failure but rather as part of the inevitable process of career development. Goals may be changed because the world is in flux, and changes in the career environment might make some goals less appealing while others become more attractive. Ideally, long-term goals help to define goals for the shorter term. If a person's career aspiration is to hold an administrative or executive position, then short-term goals should be defined in a way that leads to increased likelihood that the long-term goal will be met. Honest, self-respecting examination of progress toward a career goal is a healthy exercise. Sometimes, it results in a realization that the goal was unrealistic or not as desirable as originally thought. It also can lead to redirecting professional activities to be sure that they are aligned with the long-term objective. Or it may lead to the realization that the long-term goal is in sight and that deliberate and timely action is needed to make it happen.

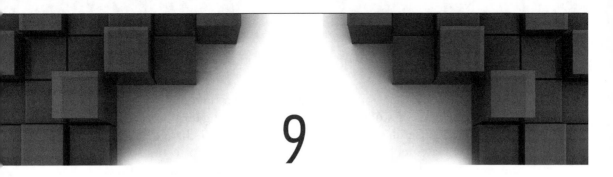

9

Long-Range Research Career Strategies

SHAPING AND MANAGING A RESEARCH PROGRAM

A beginning faculty member or newly independent scientist needs to develop strategies to meet their career goals. An excellent resource, particularly for the basic scientist, is the handbook *Making the Right Moves* (Bonetta, 2006) which can be downloaded free of charge online (http://www.hhmi.org/resources/labmanagement/downloads/moves2.pdf). Although career goals are likely to be adapted along the way, it is best to take early steps to establish clear long-term goals and identify a path for achieving those goals. Developing a clear mission statement for a laboratory helps organize a research program into a series of specific goals. That mission will help guide decisions about the research program, recruit students, and attract new staff.

Developing a Mission Statement

The mission statement should be broad, that is, a 10-year goal. Specific goals to achieve the mission should also be identified. Starting with a long-range goal, such as preventing the development of a disease, the goal can be used to lay out the necessary steps to form a research program. The goal then will be broken down into a series of aims that involve individual research studies and form the first application for research funding. In the example above, the risk factors to be considered might include genetic mutations and interactive factors such as gene regulation, environmental toxins, or injuries. Each will need to be investigated both individually and in interaction with each other. These can be aims of studies that all lead to the long-term goal. Planning for 5 to 10 years is useful, although directions likely will change along the way. The mission statement certainly is useful as a roadmap to the scientist who composes it, but it also provides direction to research staff and students.

Investing in Technology

The tendency of a new faculty member is to replicate the laboratory where they recently completed a postdoctoral fellowship. This is not always the best approach and can hinder the development of an independent research career. Certainly, some aspects of a laboratory may be replicated but a new laboratory should be moving forward into other technologies or hybrids of different approaches depending on the research goals.

One of the first needs is to be innovative in a research program; certainly a replication of the research program and research techniques from a previous laboratory won't lend itself to innovation. The key is to look outward and forward, not just backward. Often, a few visits to laboratories using new and different techniques could be time well spent before deciding on a particular direction and using all of the start-up resources in the first year. A new laboratory must use state of the art technology. Sometimes workshops are held at scientific meetings on new techniques. Other strategies are to do literature searches on new techniques. Arranging for a telephone call with an investigator using the technology or making a visit to a laboratory with new technology can be invaluable. By visiting and asking members of the laboratory about debugging issues, if measurement accuracy has been demonstrated, and how stable and reliable the techniques are is important before investing in new methods. If the staff are spending an inordinate amount of time working out the measurement issues rather than doing research, it is a good indication that the technology may not be ready to adopt. A new faculty member can't afford to devote too much time to developing new technology rather than moving ahead with their research program.

Initial Funding Strategies

A new faculty member can obtain initial support for their first study usually from internal funding and having a well-designed specific project that is ready to submit the first semester is invaluable. This will help you obtain pilot data and publish before the first grant application to an external funding source. An initial introductory visit to the Office of Sponsored Research in the first few weeks on campus can help identify initial funding support mechanisms and deadlines.

A possible first step is to find foundation funding, but this only pays off if your research closely matches the goals of a foundation. Often these are much more specific to a particular disease or population need than federal or state agencies. Searching for a foundation can be done online (http://foundation center.org/); many institutions are subscribers. The Office of Sponsored Programs or Grant and Contracts Office usually can assist with access as there is a subscription fee; however, this is low for individuals at nonprofit institutions. Subscribing to the National Institutes of Health Guide to Grants and Contract will allow you to receive alerts to new Requests for Proposals and Program Announcements and is easy and free (http://grants.nih.gov/grants/guide/listerv.htm).

A foundation grant can be a good initial start but many do not provide institutional support (that is, indirect funds), making such awards less popular to administrators. Contacting a foundation to inquire about their specific program areas is important; these are usually very specific and it could be waste of time to submit if your research interests are not a close match to those of a particular foundation.

BUILDING AND EXPANDING A RESEARCH PROGRAM

A new tenure track junior faculty member must identify and focus their research so that they are productive and quickly become recognized as making a contribution to their field, which is essential to being granted tenure. Initially, it is important to have one main focus for research, although it can be wise to eventually develop two closely related areas, one less risky than the other. Persons in basic research may have a basic research area and a translational project that relates to a disease. A "translational" basic research project may be an animal model or a cell line that is a model for a disease. On the other hand, clinical investigators may focus on a particular disease or disorder. Determining the pathogenesis may be a first step toward preventing the development of a disorder. This may require determining the factors that are involved in the development of the disorder, leading back to more basic research.

As the scientist becomes established they may want to establish two lines of research to allow them more opportunities for funding. This also allows the scientist to achieve a balance of high and moderate risk in their research so that their entire career is not invested in one area. A danger can be that if a scientist only investigates one area and that proves unsuccessful, then the scientist needs to start over from scratch. Alternatively, with two areas of research, if others beat them on achieving a research goal or their research hits a dead end, the scientist has another option for obtaining funding. It can be good to have a second area as a backup.

BECOMING A SUPERVISOR AND HIRING STAFF

Selecting good students and staff to work in your research program is essential to your success. Doctoral students and graduate students often are eager to obtain research experience and will volunteer to work in your laboratory. Such assistance can be very helpful but caution is needed before you agree to take on a doctoral student or hire staff. Many experienced scientists agree that selecting doctoral students and hiring staff can be one of the most important aspects of being a good manager; often, personality and work habits are as important as intelligence, creativity, and hard work in selecting new members of the research team.

A letter of reference usually includes only positive comments and omits the negative ones so a follow-up telephone call can sometimes prevent future problems by checking with the person on any negatives they can identify concerning a candidate. Many supervisors are reluctant to include the negative comments in a letter of reference but will be more forthright on the telephone. Most laboratories are a small group of individuals who work closely together as a research team. If one person is negative and difficult to deal with, the others will become less eager to participate; the morale of the group will suffer, and the research can be jeopardized as a result. Avoiding those who have difficulties in dealing with others, have problems sharing with others, do not accept direction, or are argumentative is essential. Asking about such characteristics when telephoning a reference can identify persons to avoid.

Positive characteristics that make for a wonderful student or staff member in a laboratory setting are those who get along well with others, are intelligent, creative, team players, sensitive to the needs to others, can take direction, are conscientious, have high ethical standards, and accept responsibility. Interviewing applicants can be highly revealing, particularly if careful thought is given in advance to the kinds of questions that are most relevant to the work responsibilities. Much can be learned from open-ended questions such as, "What would you do if [insert a difficult situation or problem, such as observing a staff member ignore calibration or test protocols, being falsely accused of neglecting a task, or being asked by someone outside the lab about confidential aspects of the research program]?" An interview is a good opportunity to learn about the applicant and also to emphasize expectations for those who work in the lab.

If a person is likely to have problems, the best approach is not to hire them or accept them into the group. Taking on a doctoral student or new staff member assumes responsibility for their actions. Being alert to poor performance or problems also requires immediate and decisive action to remedy the problems, giving feedback to persons, and giving them direction and an opportunity to remedy the problems. If they don't improve, taking action is important to prevent a negative impact on the rest of the group. The negative impact of a poor staff member or student may reflect poorly on the leader if it is not solved. The group may begin to question the leader's judgment if they do not deal with a poorly performing member of the research team. The toxic effects of a troublesome staff member or student can have long-term consequences. Avoiding hiring such a person in the first place is best; but removing them quickly once problems develop is recommended. Often, a trial period for a student is advisable before committing to being their advisor.

THE RESEARCHER AS A LEADER

Scientists have different leadership styles; some tend to micromanage, while others tend to have a hands-off style. In the former situation, micromanaging a laboratory allows members too little opportunity for having responsibility and as a result they leave everything to the laboratory director and take on little responsibility themselves. Conversely, when lab directors are too hands-off and not involved, junior members of the laboratory can take over some of the decision-making roles. Then, if problems develop it is difficult for the laboratory director to intervene when they become aware of difficulties. Both extremes can have complications; it is best when there is a more moderate level of involvement. Regular lab meetings are essential and individual meetings often are a good way to start; then, as members become more skilled and are able to take responsibility, the meetings can become less frequent.

Leadership training is now being offered to scientists and faculty in many institutions; this can be invaluable early in a scientist's career to prevent difficulties and determine how to motivate members of the research lab. Many leadership skills can be learned and these can have career-long benefits. A lab director needs to maintain a leadership role, but not be too authoritarian. Members of the laboratory may resent an authoritarian style and this can result in an uncomfortable atmosphere within the laboratory. On the other hand, the lab director shouldn't become too personally involved with the students and staff members of the lab. Although a laboratory director who becomes "a member of the gang" may enjoy working closely with their students and staff as colleagues, when difficult decisions have to be made to cut costs if funding is reduced, a sense of betrayal may develop when the laboratory director becomes more authoritarian.

Therefore, the ideal laboratory director shows respect for each member of the laboratory, but maintains some distance in order to play a decision-making role when necessary. The laboratory director should be careful to treat members equally and when members show they are able to take responsibility, give them some role in running the laboratory but checking in with them regularly to keep things on track. Group discussions are invaluable at weekly lab meetings and everyone should feel free to voice their opinions on matters although it should be recognized that the laboratory director has the final say. Of course, not getting embroiled in disputes or taking sides when two laboratory members are having differences is important. Avoiding problems is usually not a solution, however, when difficulties develop. Rather, dealing with those having difficulties in a frank and straightforward manner is important. Postponing decisions when choices need to be made also can be devastating as everyone may be uncomfortable until some direction is taken.

Some laboratories have periodic (annual) "retreats" where members can share ideas, stay tuned to the long-term goals of the project, and develop a sense of unity with others. Leading these retreats takes planning and skill. It can be helpful to review each retreat, to determine what worked well and what did not.

LABORATORY POLICIES
(ESTABLISHING STANDARD OPERATING PROCEDURES)

A laboratory chief is responsible for adherence to safety regulations of the institution in a laboratory. In a clinical research program, patient safety and confidentiality are of paramount importance, and strict adherence to the procedures and policies established by the Internal Review Board is essential. In laboratories involving animal research, research protocols approved by the Institutional Animal Care and Use Committee must be followed and amendments submitted and approved before changes are made in the research. This is equally important in clinical research programs where research protocols approved by the Internal Review Board must be followed closely and amendments submitted and approved to prevent protocol violations.

Standard operating procedure (SOP) manuals (Table 9–1) should be written and developed both for delineating roles and responsibilities but also are essential for training any new members arriving in the laboratory. A list of reading and training requirements that are checked off by new members ensures that everyone receives the necessary training. New members should

Table 9–1. Items Covered by Laboratory Standard Operating Procedures

Item	Regulations	Items Covered
Safety regulations	Institutional Safety Policies	Wearing safety glasses
		Wearing lab coats
		Wearing gloves
		Storing chemicals
		Use of a hood
		Storing flammables
		Disposal of biological waste and chemicals

Table 9–1. *continued*

Item	Regulations	Items Covered
Using Animals in Research	Institutional Animal Care and Use Committee (IACUC) NIH regulations for Use of Animals in Research Department of Agriculture	Animal protocols Animal transport Animal housing Survival surgery
Clinical Research	Internal Review Board (IRB) U.S. Department of Health and Human Services (DHHS)— Office of Human Protection from Research Risks	Clinical research protocols Protecting patient confidentiality
Ethical Practices and Research Integrity	U.S. DHHS—Office of Research Integrity	Integrity of research records and data, misconduct, Falsification, fabrication and plagiarism Authorship, peer review Conflicts of interest, mentorship
Computer use and security	Institutional policies on computer use and security U.S. DHHS Regulations covering The Health Insurance Portability and Accountability Act of 1996 (HIPAA) Privacy and Security Rules Privacy Act	Encryption of computer and storage media, HIPAA compliant secure servers for the storage and use of clinical research information
Ordering Equipment and Supplies	Institutional purchasing policy and procedures Inventory tracking of Property and Assets Budgetary authority, Auditing procedures	Responsibility for checking supplies Ordering procedures Maintaining budget and purchasing records for separate accounts
Travel Policies	Institutional policies for travel authorization and reimbursement	Procedures for requesting preapproval Per diem and lodging rates Air travel Mileage reimbursement

be given manuals on SOPs, copies of the animal and patient research protocols, and required to read them. They should be asked to sign a note saying that they have read the material and agree to follow the procedures. In this way all lab members are made responsible for following the required procedures and aware of the policies. If lab members violate policies or procedures then they can be held responsible if the laboratory director has already made certain that they are informed or the rules and procedures to be followed.

Documentation

Most institutions have rules that must be followed regarding the recording of research procedures and maintaining research records. Laboratory notebooks usually remain the property of the institution and the laboratory. Although departing staff may take copies of their notes and data with them, the originals must remain at the home institution. As records become electronic, that is when a laboratory moves to an electronic laboratory notebook (ELN) system, safeguards for having everyone participate and maintaining such records need to be developed. In clinical research, patient procedures must be recorded and confidentiality guarded through digital data encryption and security measures. It is the responsibility of the laboratory director to train and educate all of the members of their laboratory on these procedures as the lab director is usually the principal investigator on the protocols and the person responsible to either the IACUC or the IRB for following good research practices.

Becoming a Mentor

Junior scientists need to develop mentorship skills. As soon as a scientist has undergraduate honors students, masters or doctoral students, or postdoctoral trainees they have responsibilities as a mentor. This includes responsibility for shaping a young scientist's career, ensuring that they receive the training they need, giving them access to leaders in the field, helping them move to good laboratories for postdoctoral training, assisting with decisions about new positions, developing networking skills, and contacting others to help them at each stage. A mentor serves as a sounding board and a guide, providing support and advice. A scientist may be a mentor for students not directly working in their lab by providing advice to young scientists in the department or institution.

MAKING CHOICES AT DIFFERENT STAGES IN A RESEARCH CAREER

As a scientist builds their career, they often need to make decisions about priorities when trying to find a good balance between their personal and family life and their scientific career. During the early childhood years, spousal sharing of parental responsibilities is paramount. Traveling to scientific meetings may need to be reduced at the time when it is important to network with others and build a reputation. Recognizing the different demands and trying to balance them may be difficult but is important.

As a scientist becomes successful, many new opportunities may present themselves. Some scientists in midcareer may decide that they will pursue other aspects of science such as inventions, patents and licensing, and venture into the commercial sector of science. These are exciting opportunities, but can be risky (and are discussed in Chapter 11). Others decide on whether to apply for administrative positions such as chair of their department, which is the first step to moving into policy-making roles that may lead to becoming a dean, institute director, or other high-level administrative positions.

As a scientist develops a reputation, they are approached by other institutions that may offer new opportunities and facilities that are attractive. The decision on whether or not to move to another institution can be a very serious one and should be carefully investigated. Often, the laboratory equipment will need to remain with the home institution and cannot go to the new institution unless it is personal property. Institutional policies vary on this issue, and some institutions permit the relocation of equipment purchased with extramural funds, particularly if the research grant is transferred to the new institution.

When approached by another institution, the first step is to go for a visit. Even if a scientist is not seeking a position at the other institution, there are several advantages: they will gain experience on what to look for, become more experienced with interviewing and negotiation, and learn about others' research by visiting. Sometimes the scientist's home institution might give them more resources if they want to keep a successful faculty member who is thinking of leaving. However, care must be taken, as once it is thought that a scientist is leaving they can lose consideration of their future needs by the home department. There are no guarantees that the additional resources will be provided, although many scientists have benefited from retention efforts. But going to this well repeatedly can offend one's colleagues and may lead the administration to view the individual as a malcontent.

As a scientist moves into leadership positions or changes career paths, new options may develop such as taking leadership positions in government and industry. No one path is successful for everyone and different people may choose alternate paths to the same long-term goal. The purpose of this chapter is to help scientists be aware of the choices that come with making these decisions.

MOVING INSTITUTIONS

Scientists often move to new institutions when new opportunities provide tangible benefits such as promotion, different work responsibilities, improved research facilities, or new collaborations. However, this decision is a difficult one, as a move will be disruptive and can delay research progress for a year or two. The positives of advancement, new facilities, and better resources need to be weighed against the disruption caused by a move. First, as the home institution often will not allow the scientist to take their equipment with them, they will need to buy equipment and set up a new laboratory. Second, some staff members may not want to move to the new institution or there may not be positions available for staff members that a principal investigator may want to bring with them.

Negotiating A Contract

The old adage that if it isn't in writing it won't be honored still stands. E-mails discussing promises have little bearing on what to expect on arrival at an institution. Only documents signed by those who have authority at the level of the dean and provost obligate an institution; the details of the offer and contract must be signed above the level of the chair to be honored. Chairmanships can change, and although those in at the level of a dean or provost may change they ensure obligation of the institution to honor the commitment. Fiscal situations often change both at state and private institutions changing budgets, and unless the institution has a commitment in writing, start-up packages can be altered, particularly in bad times.

Taking a year before moving institutions will allow for as smooth a transition as possible; although moves are never easy. A schedule of tasks for moving can make the process easier (Figure 9–1). This will allow time for construction of new facilities to be completed well in advance of arrival. Sorting out what equipment can be moved, taking inventory of everything, and arranging for the move will take time. Ordering the new purchases and having them installed and set up before arrival at the new institution can reduce start-up time. Those involved in clinical and animal research can write their research protocols in advance and have them reviewed and approved before they arrive to reduce delays. Finally, and very importantly, by announcing the move well in advance, staff and students can plan either their own relocation or find another position at their home institution in advance of the lab move.

UPDATING TECHNOLOGY

A research program must be state of the art to compete successfully for research funds. The enhanced emphasis on innovation as a criterion in the scientific review categories for grant proposals at the National Institutes of Health make it imperative that a research program is constantly being upgraded to using state of the art techniques. However, great care must be taken in knowing when to move into new techniques. It can be tempting to want to acquire a new technology before others but you may waste time working out the bugs while losing momentum in your research by having to dedicate too much

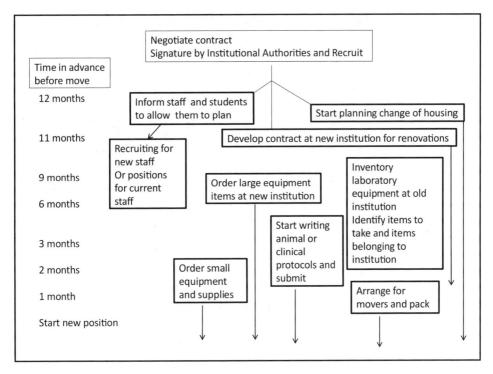

FIGURE 9–1. Planning and executing an institutional move.

time to demonstrating the validity and reliability of a new technology. The dangers of being involved in the beta phase of the development of new technology can be particularly precarious for a new investigator. New investigators trying to establish themselves are at a disadvantage if they also are trying to prove a new technology at the same time. The new technology may still need to be worked out, and may distract a new investigator from developing their research program.

Adoption of new technology is a matter of timing. If you are one of the first to use it, you cannot be certain of whether or not it will meet your needs and you could waste valuable time on a technique that may never bear fruit. It is best to let others do the very early development and wait until they have worked out the bugs before adopting it. Although using state of the art techniques is important, caution must be used not to risk wasting time on something that may never work. Second, you may need to demonstrate that it is both valid and reliable to grant reviewers. Although federal agencies want you to be innovative, at the same time the reviewers must accept the methods you are using as valid and reliable and state of the art. If you are too far ahead of the curve they won't give you the benefit of the doubt and consider the application too risky for funding. Often, the best time to pick up a new technology is just after it becomes commercially available. A company has determined that there is a market for the technology and that they can manufacture or produce it in a stable and reliable fashion.

Taking on Administrative Responsibilities

As a scientist progresses in their research career they can be offered promotions and new positions, usually as a director of a research center or a chair of a department. Here, management style is very important and the hiring of good administrative support staff is essential to success. The administrative assistant is the most important person to a director or chair. They must be organized, able to multitask, strong enough to protect their director from constant interruptions, reliable, able to maintain confidentiality about personnel matters and budget, and trustworthy. As a director for a center or department, a careful balance must be maintained between allowing faculty or scientists at the center to participate in decision-making so that they buy in to any new directions being taken but at the same time decisions need to be reached in order to move forward.

Becoming a Senior Investigator

This stage in a career often occurs without announcement, but as invitations to give keynote addresses at large international meetings increase and honor awards are received, the status of being a leader in the field becomes evident and there are responsibilities that come with that status. Being on panels setting research priorities for foundations, writing review articles for journals about future research directions, serving on Advisory Councils to Institutes at the National Institutes of Health, chairing Study Sections, and reviewing applicants for tenure at universities are some of the added responsibilities that come with being a leader in a field. Such leadership roles are important for assuring that the future of one's discipline continues with new investigators establishing new laboratories and exciting new avenues of research. In clinical research, the need to address patient care and to have rapid transfer of research findings to clinical application is of paramount importance.

Retirement or Changing Careers

Finally, the issues of retirement emerge, a critical decision. Some persons take on new careers in policy-making positions while others assume part-time positions, consulting, or transfer to Professor Emeritus which can allow use of the institutions' facilities and being available to junior faculty and graduate students on a voluntary basis. Transferring to a new position such as policy making at a federal agency can be very invigorating as a scientist's knowledge and experience can be put to good use. Second careers are becoming more frequent. Many persons who have been bench scientists until they reach mid/late career may then take training to become a health scientist administrator at the National Institutes of Health, either as a member of program staff or as a scientific review officer.

When considering retirement, some scientists continue to be productive well into their seventies and retire later. However, if one is no longer productive and remains in a tenured position it is important not to linger too long. By staying, an unproductive professor may be preventing the department from recruiting new faculty to develop new areas of research. It is embarrassing when senior members constantly feel the need to comment at meetings when their remarks are no longer of high importance. Knowing when to leave is important and bowing out gracefully allows a senior investigator to continue to be held in high regard by others. Scientists develop friendships with colleagues often throughout the world and it is important to maintain those friendships after retirement. Continuing to attend meetings allows one to maintain such friendships and visit with friends and colleagues in a more leisurely fashion.

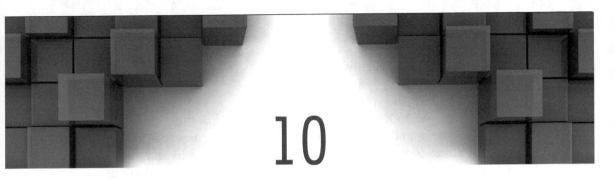

10

Achieving Success in Academia

*I*n its issue of July 13, 2008, *U.S. News & World Report* selected *professor* as one of the 31 best careers for the year. This news item is an encouraging introduction to a chapter on a career in academia. The article went on to point out some positive, and some not so positive, aspects of the academic life. Classroom hours of 6 to 15 hours per week were considered a protection against burnout, and the atmosphere of a college campus was viewed as a definite attraction. One negative aspect was the uncertainty of getting a tenure-track faculty position. There are positive and negative features beyond those noted in the magazine article. One aspect of academia that many find appealing is the challenge of discovering and disseminating knowledge, and in most cases, considerable freedom in designing the path to knowledge discovery. On the negative side, educational preparation for an academic position requires 5 to 8 years beyond the baccalaureate, not including postdoctoral study, which is common in many disciplines. During their education, many students take on a substantial debt. Once the PhD is earned, there is no guarantee that a suitable position will be available, although demand for professors varies widely across specialties. For that matter, professorial lives vary widely as well. This chapter attempts to paint a general picture of what a professor does and how achievements in academia are rewarded through promotion and the hallowed status of tenure.

THE BIG THREE OF A PROFESSOR'S WORKLOAD

A senior faculty member at the University of Wisconsin-Madison once said that promotion to associate professor with tenure was based on three things: research, research, research. He probably made this comment only partly in jest. But as important as research may be to promotion in many universities, most academics work hard to achieve a balance across three major areas—teaching, research, and service. This trinity is nearly universal in the documents that are used to support promotion and tenure. And jokes aside, most faculty members are keenly interested in teaching and willingly do their duties in the service category.

One of the biggest challenges that a new faculty member confronts is time management. A recent survey showed that the number one cause of stress for young faculty is balancing the time needed for teaching and research (Berberet, 2008). The first year of a faculty appointment is particularly challenging because of the confluence of demands that include course preparation, setting up a research program, writing grant applications, and serving on department or university committees. The pressure of this period should not be underestimated, but it is good to remember that things usually get easier. Typically, a faculty member does not have to prepare new courses every year, as at least some of the courses are offered repeatedly. Therefore, the investment in course preparation during the first year of a faculty appointment pays dividends that are realized when the courses are taught again in the future. But it is probably true that time management and the pressure of meeting multiple demands continue as career-long challenges for most academics.

TEACHING

Let's take a closer look at the beginning of an academic career to get a sense of the demands and priorities that must be addressed, beginning with teaching. Many newly hired faculty members will receive teaching relief in the form of a reduced teaching load for their first term or even the first year. This is important when negotiating a favorable start-up package that includes teaching relief in the first year and sometimes in the third year before the first review. The reduced teaching obligation can be extremely helpful, as it not only reduces the time needed for the overall instructional effort but it enables the faculty member to focus on a smaller number of courses to develop effective teaching materials. Many new faculty members are taken by surprise by the time needed to prepare lectures, laboratory sessions, examinations, and related items (e.g., handouts, Web-based supplements, and makeup examinations). It is a common experience to discover that teaching can take as much time as one wants to give to it. But, of course, faculty members cannot devote all of their time to teaching. There are other masters to serve, and they make strong demands on time and energy. By virtue of the academic calendar and schedule of courses, teaching is one of the most consistent activities in a professor's life. Lectures must be prepared, classes must be met, and exams must be given. The regularity of the demands requires a commensurate regularity in time management. Students are not inclined to forgive a sloppy or negligent lecture. Course evaluations usually include feedback that is to the point.

Even some of the fundamental aspects of teaching can seem difficult at first. New faculty members often find that they are not successful in predicting how much material can be covered in a class period. Sometimes, the class period outlasts the instructional material, but at other times, the class period ends before even half of the material has been presented. Both outcomes can be frustrating and can undo the intentions expressed in the course syllabus. It can help greatly to rehearse lectures to get some indication of how long it will take to cover the planned materials. Rehearsal has other benefits as well, such as promoting the flow of ideas and natural transitions between topics.

Another challenge is packaging information so that it is readily absorbed by students. In their zeal to be informative, new faculty sometimes barrage students with detailed information that is not effectively structured to reflect the main questions or ideas. Effective teaching requires a constant eye on the main goals of instruction. It is key to remember that, even when an instructor believes the goals are clear, students who are unfamiliar with the material may not share this belief. Beginning and ending a lecture with the main ideas can help students to develop a mental framework for organizing and understanding the information they receive.

There is no single style of teaching that works for everyone. Certainly, there are some basic recommendations and cautions that are nearly universal, but each faculty member has a unique personality and a unique combination of strengths and weaknesses. It can sometimes help to model ourselves after successful teachers we have had, but this does not always yield the desired results. Teaching day after day and year after year provides the experience from which teaching style can be developed and refined. Very few faculty members, even those with years of experience in the classroom, feel satisfied that every lecture they give meets their internal standards of success.

The preceding comments use the concept of lecturing as convenient shorthand for instructional activities. But contemporary teaching involves much more than lecturing, although lectures continue as the centerpiece of instruction in most campuses. Teaching often includes a menu of instructional methods, with increasing reliance on technologies such as Web-based instruction, distance education, and so on. Some resources are listed in Appendix 10A, but the list is by no means exhaustive of the wealth of information that is available on this topic.

It is now routine procedure in most institutions of higher learning for faculty to be evaluated by students, usually in the form of a written evaluation that may or may not be standardized within the institution. This is a major change that has come about in 4 or 5 decades. In the 1960s, it was rare for professors to be evaluated by the students they taught. This is not to say that student evaluations are the only way by which teaching can or should be assessed. Appendix 10B lists several different forms of evaluation. Although using all of these methods may be prohibitive in terms of time and effort, some combination probably is the best way to assess education in a way that is informative and unbiased.

RESEARCH AND SCHOLARSHIP

Accomplishments in research and scholarship are an integral part of academic life in most colleges and universities. The actual expectations differ across universities, and it is risky to make any general statements regarding faculty performance in terms of numbers and types of publications, or size and type of research grants and contracts. Research productivity is important not only for promotion within the original hiring institution, but also for potential moves to another institution. In addition, many faculty members derive considerable satisfaction from their research and from the resulting publications.

It is not easy to generalize about research. It takes many different forms and accommodates many different work patterns. But a few general statements can be made. First, research is demanding of both time and care. Cutting corners is risky to the point of career suicide. Data are earned through dedicated effort, and scientific integrity rides on the care that is taken during every stage of a research project. Second, research is fully valued only when it is disseminated. Data stored in a file or computer memory mean little to anyone other than the investigator unless and until they are made generally available in a scientific journal or other outlet. Third, research requires a mindset that continually seeks understanding of the problem at hand. It draws on resources such as the published literature and discussions with colleagues and students. If professors can seem like self-absorbed pedants at times, it may be because of their dedication to the pursuit of understanding.

Research fuels two things that bring prestige and influence to universities: publications and grants (or contracts). Publications announce accomplishments to the world, and grants are the economic drive that ensures a vital research program. As important as teaching is, the reputation of a successful teacher rarely goes beyond the campus boundaries, but articles published in a premier journal attract attention to both the authors and to their affiliated institution. No surprise then that a college or university that wants to promote its reputation may look first at the potential to enhance its research productivity. And nothing succeeds like success. Publications are the best evidence that an academic can deliver on the promise of scientific or scholarly discovery. Extramural funds (i.e., monies from outside agencies such as the federal government, state government, or private groups) are the capital on which universities depend to support research.

There has long been an interest in developing a metric that accounts for research productivity and quality—for journals, academic units, and individual scientists. Some metrics are being used for important decisions, such as the granting of tenure, so it is important to know something about how these numbers are generated.

The journal impact factor, reported by Journal Citation Report (JCR), is a product of Thomson ISI (Institute for Scientific Information). The intent of the journal impact factor is to provide an index of the frequency with which the "average article" in a journal has been cited in a given period of time, usually 3 years. Papers that are published in journals with a high journal impact factor may be helpful in promotion and tenure decisions. Therefore, this index is one factor to consider in deciding where a scientific paper should be submitted.

Metrics also have been proposed for individual scientists. An advantage of the h-index is that it combines an assessment of both quantity (number of papers) and quality (impact, or citations to these papers) (Glänzel, 2006). To achieve a high h-index, a scientist must publish a fairly large number of papers which then must be cited by other scientists. As in the case of the journal impact factor, quality is measured by frequency of citation. An advantage of the h-index over some other possible metrics is that it guards against the biasing effect of a single article that has a substantial number of citations. It also has an obvious advantage over metrics that recognize only the total number of papers published, with no regard to their impact.

At the department, school, or university level, another index has been adopted by a growing number of institutions—the Faculty Scholarly Productivity Index™ (FSP Index) is designed for the evaluation of doctoral programs at research universities (across all Carnegie research classifications). The index is derived from a set of statistical algorithms using data on several categories of faculty productivity, including publications (books and journal articles), citations of journal publications, federal research funding, and awards and honors.

Is impact in the sense of frequency of citation a true reflection of quality? Perhaps not, but the fact that it is fairly easily quantified from publication data seems sufficient to ensure its use. Numbers convey a sense of objectivity, especially when the numbers are based on simple counts. But frequency of citation varies with scientific specialty. The greater the number of scientists working in a particular area, the larger is the potential citation frequency of their papers.

SERVICE

Service is a cover term for the manifold activities that faculty members perform to keep academic departments and units operational. Committee service is a major part of this role, but it also can include student advising and mentoring; service to local, state, and federal agencies, service to professional organizations; involvement with other educational agencies; reviewing research articles and grants; and still other activities. Universities are not completely uniform as to how the service category is defined. For example, reviewing journal articles and grant applications could also be considered as falling under the research and scholarship category.

Typically, service is given the least weight of the teaching/research/service triad in decisions regarding promotion and tenure. Many universities assign weightings of 40% teaching, 40% research, and 20% service. Rarely would service be the paramount factor in a promotion leading to tenure. But this is not to say that service is negligible. An important part of citizenship in the academic community is to help shoulder the administrative and committee obligations. Moreover, participation in service roles can help to shape the future of a department, college or school, or the university itself.

Service is a way to learn about how a college or university works. Through committee service, new faculty members can learn about institutional policy, chains of command, cross-departmental relations, and the means to effect change. This is not say that everyone relishes committee assignments, and there are some who avoid committee service whenever possible. But such avoidance comes at the risk of alienating faculty colleagues who must cover the debt in service workload that is created when a faculty member does not take his or her share.

With seniority, the service load usually increases, often substantially so. Tenured faculty are called on not only to serve as chair for committees in their own departments, but they also may be appointed to divisional or college committees, internal review boards, and other transdepartmental committees and boards. Some will chair their departments, and a few will move to positions in higher administration, such as dean, director, provost, or chancellor. One of the most important responsibilities of tenured professors is to mentor and evaluate untenured faculty. This duty, along with the responsibility to recruit new assistant professors to the department, means that tenured faculty members design the department's future in substantial ways.

THE CURRICULUM VITAE

A curriculum vitae (singular), is from Latin and means "course of one's life." It is often abbreviated as CV or simply called a "vita." The curriculum vitae is a document that describes in some detail an individual's academic and professional accomplishments. Curricula vitae (plural) are typically used for academic or research positions. Resumes are similar documents that summarize work experience and education and are used in business and industry. The CV is a reflection of achievement and it is important that it be accurate and reasonably complete. Generally, CVs are much longer than resumes, especially for individuals with a long career. Appendix 10C lists some of the categories that are used in forming a CV, but this is by no means a system that should be rigidly and uniformly applied. The major consideration is that the CV provides a coherent and transparent record of important accomplishments. The CV grows in number of pages as a career grows in length and achievement. It is not simply a matter of adding items under categories, but also a matter of adding categories to maintain a satisfactory account of career contributions. Giving thought to the form of a CV is well worth the effort to a newly hired assistant professor. Ideally, the CV should lend itself to easy updating, and it should convey the individual's accomplishments in a clear and honest manner. CVs should document efforts in teaching, research, and service, but they should avoid "fluff" or self-congratulation.

Often, it is useful, although somewhat more work, to maintain different types of CVs. There is the traditional NIH Biosketch which focuses on area of expertise, positions, honors, peer-reviewed publications, and external funding received. This has recently been altered to be changed to listing only 15 peer-reviewed journal publications; five related to the topic of the grant application, five most recognized publications (in highest impact journals or most cited), and five most recent. A more complete CV is usually needed for a tenure review, listing courses taught, theses directed, and in addition to refereed journal publications and external funding, also includes nonrefereed publications such as books and book chapters and invited national and international lectures and keynote addresses. A CV for applying for jobs will depend on whether it is a scientific position, academic, or both on whether teaching is included. Most CVs include the items listed in Appendix 10C.

One rule is to never list articles as "in preparation," most institutions only consider articles that are published or "in press," after the letter of acceptance for publication has been received. "Epub" articles should be included. Articles "under review" usually are not included as they may be rejected at any time.

THE NEW FACULTY MEMBER: PREPARED FOR WHAT?

Legion is the number of assistant professors who measure themselves against the challenges of a professorial life only to conclude that they are not adequately prepared. A recent survey (Berberet, 2008) bears this out. When asked to gauge their level of preparation for various activities, the percentage of respondents indicating that they were very effectively prepared was: conduct research (33%), teach undergraduates (31%), interdisciplinary collaboration (25%), teach using technology (20%), articulate teaching philosophy (19%), serve on faculty committees (10%), advise undergraduates (8%), and obtain grants (7%). No more than one-third of the respondents judged themselves as very effective in the major domains of academic work! That may not seem a satisfying self-assessment. Obviously, a great deal of on the job learning must occur if these junior members of the faculty are to have a more positive judgment of their competence. It is no shame to feel "green" when embarking on a faculty position, and one should not feel that everyone else is better prepared. The simple fact of the matter is that most doctoral programs are not designed to prepare students to be highly competent in all these roles. Rather, doctoral training provides a basic level of knowledge and experience that should enable the newly minted doctorate to enter the academic workforce and rapidly build the required expertise. This comment is not meant to say that higher education is immune to criticism. To the contrary, recent reports indicate that there is a good deal that could be done to improve doctoral education.

POSTDOCTORAL STUDIES

In many academic fields, but especially the physical and biological sciences, it is commonplace to do postdoctoral study before landing a faculty position, and in some fields two postdoctoral placements are now becoming commonplace. Such a study provides excellent opportunities to learn or refine research skills, publish papers, learn the finer points of research grant applications, and explore possible steps for career development. Postdoctoral study is discussed in Chapter 1.

THE PROMOTIONAL LADDER AND TENURE

Faculty ranks vary somewhat across institutions, but the prevailing system recognizes three ranks of professorship: assistant, associate, and full. Most newly recruited faculty members begin at the assistant professor level, which can be on a tenure track or not. Tenure track means that the individual has the potential to earn tenure, which usually comes at the same time as promotion to associate professor. It is important to note that some faculty positions are not on the tenure track. A position description should be very clear on this point, and, if it is not, it is wise to ask about it.

TENURE—THE WHAT AND WHY

Although tenure has been an important aspect of academia, it is not without controversy. Tenure is a way of protecting faculty members from loss of their positions if they take unpopular positions on an issue, or if they criticize government officials. Therefore, tenure helps to ensure academic freedom. But it also can be viewed as a form of job security, in which the granting of tenure is assurance that the holder of tenure is not likely to be dismissed from a position, barring extraordinary financial circumstances in the employing institution or personal conduct that is unacceptable to the community at large.

Critics of tenure claim that it can lead to academic deadwood—professors who no longer have to demonstrate productivity to keep their jobs. However, most universities have developed systems of posttenure review in which tenured professors are reviewed at regular intervals.

Tenure is surrounded by philosophical and policy debates that are not likely to end soon. Despite continued, and sometimes harsh, criticism, tenure remains a fixture of professorial life in most academic institutions. Carmichael (1988) explained the preservation of tenure on the principle that worker-professors play a fundamental role in selecting new members of the academy. To illustrate this concept, Carmichael compared the employment methods used in baseball and universities. In baseball, the owners, working through their agents, decide which players will be assigned to a position on the team. This is an example of owner management. In academe, the incumbent worker-professors have a major responsibility to select new faculty members and to determine the positions they will assume. Academe therefore is an example of labor management.

It is important to consider why tenure persists in the face of biting criticism from those outside (and sometimes inside) the academy. Tenure is virtually unknown in other professions—physicians, attorneys, dentists, and pharmacists make no claim to it. So why is tenure central to career advancement in higher education? What would happen if it were abandoned? One way of answering these questions is to examine the life of academics in parts of the world where tenure is virtually unknown. Europe is a good place for us to make this inquiry. According to an article in *Science* (Wald, 2008), many European academics covet the tenure system of their American counterparts, for the reason that career structures in Europe vary across nations and generally offer little in the way of job security. For example, an academic in Europe may work on a research project for 5 years with little confidence that the project (and employment) will continue after that period.

In the United States and Canada, assistant professors are usually hired for renewable contract terms of 2 or 3 years. If they perform satisfactorily, then their positions will be renewed, up to 7 years. Promotion to associate professor and tenure must occur by the sixth year or termination will result. This is the basis for the notorious "up or out year," in which the individual is either promoted or leaves the institution (and sometimes academia altogether). The "tenure clock" has 7 hours on its face, and it starts ticking the moment an assistant professor starts working on contract. Getting tenure is a reward for meritorious accomplishment, and it carries great benefits. It is the holy grail of the academic.

The importance of the "up or out year" should not eclipse the importance of earlier milestones. Some assistant professors never get beyond 3 or 4 years in a department, because their contracts were not renewed after a 3-year review. That is, departments often will conduct a thorough review of an assistant professor's progress well before an actual tenure decision is made. Assistant professors who are judged not to be making satisfactory progress may be terminated as the result of this review. Therefore, it is extremely important for an assistant professor to develop a work plan that is geared to the department's expectations for promotion to tenure. It is risky business to assume that productivity in the fourth, fifth, or sixth year of an academic appointment will ensure a tenured position. Progress should be carefully planned and documented for each year of an initial appointment. Fortunately, the assistant professor usually does not have to walk through this process without sage counsel. Senior faculty colleagues generally will advise assistant professors on the march toward tenure, as discussed in the next section.

MENTORS AND MENTORING COMMITTEES

Increasingly, universities appoint mentors or mentoring committees to support and advise assistant professors on tenure tracks. The mentoring role can be very helpful, but there surely is a considerable variation in the quality of advice given. It behooves the untenured assistant professor to work closely with the mentor or mentoring committee, and to show good faith in responding to their suggestions. With few exceptions, senior members of the faculty want junior members to succeed. After all, a failed tenure decision can reflect poorly on the recruitment process by which new faculty come to the department. The first step of tenure approval is at the department level, and it is at this step that the concept of labor management by worker-professors is most evident. Typically, the tenure decision must be approved by higher authorities, such as a cross-departmental divisional committee and the dean of the college or school.

TENURE—AN EARLY CHAPTER, NOT A FINAL ONE

Tenure is justly celebrated as a major milestone in the academic life. Not only does it convey a coveted form of job security, but it also marks a professional maturity that can open the door to new opportunities (and more work!). The tenured associate professor is more likely than the untenured assistant professor to chair department committees, supervise student research projects, be appointed to cross-departmental university committees, mentor new faculty, and take on responsibilities in professional societies. Professors often discover that promotion to a tenured rank does not mean a reduced workload, but quite the opposite. Tenure may bestow a sense of security but not necessarily a reduction in hours worked. As individual faculty members take on the tenure challenge, the broader issues underlying tenure as a key aspect of professorial privilege can be eclipsed by the anxieties and pressures felt by men and women who run the gauntlet of academic review. The rationale for tenure should be explained, debated, and defended.

THE MUCH EXAMINED LIFE OF A PROFESSOR

Academics are under continual scrutiny. Manuscripts submitted for publication in refereed journals means that other scientists will examine the paper closely and may occasionally be harsh in their judgment. Research grant applications usually are subject to peer review. Teaching is evaluated by students, with results published online for the world to see. Thin skins do not serve well in academia. The scrutiny is intense for those seeking tenure, but granting of tenure does not spell an end to it. Post-tenure reviews, peer reviews of publications and grants, and teaching evaluations ensure that professors will face a career-long examination of their professional contributions. Departmental reputations depend on the efforts of all faculty, tenured and nontenured.

LIFE BALANCE

To this point, just about everything that has been said relates to work in the academic life. But work itself must be balanced against the other things in life, including family, friends, relaxation, exercise, and personal pursuits such as hobbies. For the most part, academics determine their own time management outside of fixed schedules for lectures, committee meetings, and other routine events. Some faculty members may work the conventional 8-hour day, but many will work during evening and weekend hours out of choice or necessity. There is a very real risk that the workload of academic life will eat up most available hours—to the detriment of family, friends, and enjoyment of life outside the office or laboratory. Faculty members often find that some of the tasks that need to be done cannot be accomplished during their office hours. So they might find themselves taking home a 300-page dissertation that must be read, 45 essay exams that have to graded, a journal article they have been asked to review for a refereed journal, or a grant application that might earn funding for a research project.

Let's take a look at a typical assistant professor. Of course, there is really no such thing as a "typical" assistant professor, but statistical information can be used to create at least a rough picture of the young academic, beginning with chronologic age. The typical age of a doctorate recipient in 2003 was 31.8 years in science and engineering, 34.6 years in the humanities, 37.2 years in health, 43.5 years in education, and 37.5 years in the "professional/other fields" category. A number of doctoral graduates pursue postdoctoral study, sometimes for as long as 4 or 5 years following the completion of their formal education. Therefore, most assistant professors are in the age decade of 30 to 40 years when they undertake their first academic appointment. Many already have started families, many carry debts accumulated during their education, and just about all of them look forward to earning a living wage and giving up at last life as a student. Our typical thirty-something assistant professor works about 51 hours per week (which is actually a little less than their later career colleagues). The way in which this work effort is divided across activities varies across departments and universities. Some may devote the lion's share to research, but for the majority, teaching is the major recipient of the junior academic's time. Every hour of classroom contact is accompanied by time needed for lecture (and sometimes laboratory) preparation, meetings with individual students, answering e-mail and conducting e-mail discussion groups, composing exams, grading exams and papers, and doing tasks associated with maintaining class rosters.

After several years of hard work and learning how to succeed in the academic life, the assistant professor may reach the all-important goal of promotion with tenure. By this time, he or she will be close to 40 years old, if not older. The next promotion would be to full professor. When this will happen is highly variable, but it is not unusual for an associate professor to labor about another decade before receiving this final promotion. In many universities, associate and full professors have about the same responsibilities. Tenure brings with it a fuller participation in managing the affairs of the department.

Let's assume that the professor in our example seeks extramural research support from NIH, and make the happy assumption that the grant application is successful. The average age of the first-time R01 equivalent investigator is 42.6 years. (See Chapter 7 for a discussion of NIH research grant types, such as the R01.) Most research grant applications request support for 5 years, which is the amount of time needed for a research project of average magnitude.

Some academics recommend family planning that takes into account such things as academic calendar, tenure decision, sabbatical eligibility, and research leaves. Although it is not always possible to design or constrain family life in accord with professional life, it is often possible to plan things in such a way that family and professional interests are happily balanced. However, given the loss of women from science as they progress through the ranks, it is now recognized that the academic and research environment need to better accommodate to the needs of women scientists to prevent the loss of the numbers of women scientists at the later stages in the research career and academic life.

WOMEN IN BIOMEDICAL RESEARCH CAREERS

The NIH and academia recently have begun to address the high dropout rate of women in biomedical research. Although women constitute close to half of the postdoctoral candidates, the percentage declines significantly through the academic ranks from assistant to associate and full professors. In 2008 a conference was convened at the NIH to address this issue and a report was published entitled, "Best Practices for Sustaining Career Success" (http://

womeninscience.nih.gov/bestpractices/docs/BestPracticesReport.pdf) providing the following major recommendations:

- Analyze programs currently being used for efficacy and "best practices"
- Secure a strong personal commitment to change from top management
- Employ open and transparent policies and processes for hiring, salary, and promotion decisions
- Reward success
- Enlarge the recruiting pools by looking at nontraditional sources
- Highlight the achievements of successful women and provide networking opportunities
- Institute "family-friendly" policies such as providing daycare services and flexible work schedules
- Look for points of commonality between women's programs and broader diversity programs
- Establish programs to address the needs of female faculty and scientists at each stage in their careers (e.g., stop the clock for childbearing during the tenure track period),
- Provide fair and equitable access to physical, financial, and organizational resources
- Include women on search committees

It is too early to determine whether institutions will adopt these suggestions and changes will occur to prevent the loss of women scientists from careers in biomedical research which is detrimental to science and society.

SABBATICALS AND STUDY LEAVES

One of the perks of academic life is the sabbatical. Not every college or university has a sabbatical program, but those that do offer a genuine opportunity for personal development. In some universities, study leaves are offered to faculty, but these are very similar to sabbaticals. The word *sabbatical* is derived from the Late Latin *sabbaticus*, from the Greek *sabbatikos*, and from the Hebrew *shabbathon* (i.e., Sabbath). The notion of a sabbatical is rooted in the Bible, which mentions several times the idea of rest or refraining from work. One example is in Leviticus 25, which commands that the fields should be allowed to rest for one year in every seven. But academic sabbaticals are not periods of rest or leisure. Rather, they are designed as times of renewal or dedication to special projects. The sabbatical is a type of human resource development, in which a member of a faculty is released from the routine duties of academia to pursue interests that are expected to increase his or her value to the employing institution. Sabbaticals are rarely given without consideration of a planned activity that is approved by the faculty and higher administration. Among the projects that may be the centerpiece of a sabbatical request are: writing a book, developing a new course or research specialty, preparing a set of multimedia materials to accompany a course, and establishing a research collaboration with scientists in another institution. Although sabbaticals are best known in academia, business corporations are realizing the benefits of sabbaticals to their employees and to the vitality of business at hand.

The convention of scheduling sabbaticals in 7-year periods may or may not say something about typical cycles of the human need for renewal. In a tongue-in-cheek editorial, Charlton (2006) suggested that scientific life should be measured in intervals of 7 years. He explains that 7 years is roughly the duration of high school education, the time spent in traditional basic training in science, and the time needed for early postdoctoral work to become an acknowledged expert.

CONCLUSION

The academic life has much to recommend it, but anyone considering a career in higher education should weigh the costs and benefits. Although many professors find their lives to be highly satisfying, others experience considerable stress and disappointment. An academic career has several unusual, if not unique, facets, including a form of labor management by which universities are operated: tenure as all-important career step, threefold work responsibilities, and sabbaticals as an opportunity for renewal and self-development.

APPENDIX 10A

Online Resources for Teaching in Colleges and Universities

1. gradschool.about.com/od/collegeteaching/Teaching_Resources_for_Professors.htm

   Links to several topics, including mentoring, preparing a syllabus, lecturing, teaching a survey course, and promoting undergraduate research in science.

2. honolulu.hawaii.edu/intranet/committees/FacDevCom/guidebk/teachtip/teachtip.htm

   Links to a number of topics, including professional ethics in teaching, course syllabus preparation, teaching techniques, course design, and critical thinking.

3. serc.carleton.edu/introgeo/interactive/howto.html

   Advice on how to give an interactive lecture that catches and maintains attention.

4. bokcenter.harvard.edu/icb/icb.do

   This site for the Derek Bok Center for Teaching and Learning has links to several topics, including: Semester planning, syllabus planning, activity-based learning, grading and feedback, course assessment, and interpreting evaluations.

5. web.mit.edu/tll/teaching-materials/index-teaching-materials.html

   This site maintained by the MIT Teaching and Learning Laboratory has links including: teaching during a health crisis (flu outbreak), contracts in the classroom, course evaluations, grading rubrics, learning objectives, strategic teaching and strategic teaching analysis, and teaching teamwork.

APPENDIX 10B

Different Forms of Teaching Evaluation (Berk, 2006)

Student ratings

Peer ratings

External expert ratings

Videos

Student interviews

Alumni ratings

Employer ratings

Administrator ratings

Teaching scholarship

Teaching awards

Learning outcome measures

Teaching portfolios

APPENDIX 10C

Major Categories to Consider in Developing and Maintaining a Curriculum Vitae

Most categories are used at the discretion of the individual, but the content should be as informative as reasonably possible.

Your Contact Information

Name

Address

Telephone

Cell phone

E-mail

Web page

Personal Information

Date of birth

Place of birth

Citizenship

Visa status

Gender

Optional Personal Information

Marital status

Spouse's name

Children

Employment History
List in chronologic order, include position details and dates

Work history

Academic positions

Research and training

Education

Include dates, majors, and details of degrees, training, and certification

High school

University

Graduate school

Postdoctoral training

Professional Qualifications

Certifications and accreditations

Computer skills

Awards and honors

Publications in journals

Books

Other publications

Invited national and international lectures and keynote addresses

Professional memberships

Interests

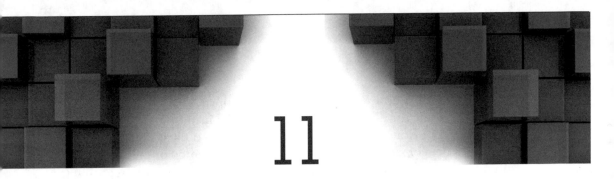

11

Technology Transfer, Patents, and Licensing

*I*ntellectual property is now an important commodity at universities and research institutions. Every institution has heard about the Gatorade story (http://www.research.ufl.edu/publications/explore/v08n1/gatorade.html). Professor Cade at the University of Florida invented the formula that became marketed as Gatorade, and since 1973 the invention has resulted in over 80 million dollars in funds being made available for research and development at the University of Florida because of royalties to the University and the inventors. Over the last 20 years most research institutions have invested funds into technology transfer in the hopes of garnering patents and licensing them to companies for the development of products that will result in royalties to the university and the inventors. As a result, most institutions now require faculty and staff to report all new inventions such as ideas for developing medical devices, new biologics, novel laboratory instruments, improved treatment methods, new drugs or agents, isolation of proteins, antibodies, and so forth. Almost all institutions now require their scientists or faculty to sign agreements when they come on board agreeing that they will report any new intellectual property or inventions to the technology transfer office.

EMPLOYEE INVENTION REPORTS

Reports of new intellectual property are filed as Employee Invention Reports (EIRs). These inventions belong to the institution unless the employee can show that they did not use institutional facilities and did the development on their own time. If the new invention was developed in a laboratory at the institution or while the scientist was working at the institution then the intellectual property belongs to the institution. The time to file an EIR is as soon as the idea is developed and long before it will be presented or published. The institution needs lead time to evaluate the potential of the invention for filing a provisional patent, the possible market, and how unique the invention is compared to other patents already awarded in the field. Once an idea is presented at a meeting it is in the public domain and is no longer patentable as it has become public knowledge. Therefore, an employee needs to give a long lead time between filing an EIR and when they plan to present or publish the idea. A 3- to 6-month lead time is needed so that a review committee can review the EIR and if the decision is made to file, time is needed for a patent attorney to be hired to work with the inventor on developing the provisional patent application.

FILING PROVISIONAL PATENTS

The first decision after the employee files the invention report is whether or not the institution plans to apply for a provisional patent on the invention. Before a provisional patent application is filed, the invention should not be divulged to anyone outside the institution; particularly companies who may recognize the commercial potential and file a provisional patent. Before submitting an abstract for a meeting, presenting new data at a meeting, or submitting a manuscript to a journal, investigators should consider whether patentable ideas are contained within the work that should be submitted as an EIR and a provisional patent filed before submission. Calling the technology transfer office regarding whether or not to file an EIR is advised.

The institution will decide whether or not to file a provisional patent based on the invention report (Figure 11–1).

This decision is not an easy one as filing even a provisional patent is costly in terms of attorney fees. Most institutions have advisory committees involved in assessing the potential of inventions for commercialization. Important issues to be considered include: the potential size of the market, the cost of development of the invention, related patents and possible overlap with those patents, and competing inventions that are already serving the same market. When filing the EIR, it is important to address each of these issues. Also, it can be beneficial to identify companies that might be interested in licensing the patent for commercial development and to demonstrate that existing patents do not overlap. If the institution is going to pay for a patent attorney to develop the application, they will need to be persuaded that the invention holds opportunity for significant income in the future to warrant the expenditure of funds beforehand. Knowing companies that already are in the market who might be interested in licensing the patent is very useful.

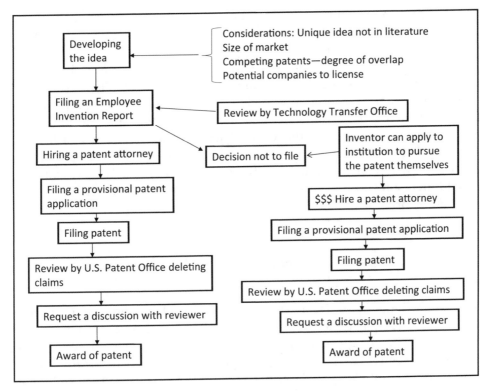

FIGURE 11–1. The patent application and award process.

Because filing a patent is an expensive process, the university or institution may decide not to pursue the invention. Then the inventor may negotiate with the institution to release the invention to allow them to pursue it with their own funds, although this happens only rarely. If the institution decides to pursue the patent, the scientist will be the inventor on the filing but they usually must assign their rights to the institution. If an invention was developed as a result of government funds, the Bayh-Dole Act applies. This was adopted by Congress in 1980, and stipulates that universities and other institutions and their inventors must be allowed to have control over their inventions even if government funds supported the development of an invention (http://www.niddk.nih.gov/patient/patent.pdf).

FILING PATENTS

The pursuit of a patent is a long and expensive process. Once a provisional patent has been filed, then the full application must be made within a year of provisional filing. After filing, the patent will take several years before a response is received from an examiner at the United States Patent Office.

The most important aspect of a filing a patent are the claims. These are listed after background information and drawings. The examiner at the patent office will review all related approved patents to make certain that none of the claims have been previously accepted. The inventor must show how these claims differ from previous claims. Also, patent examiners may designate some claims as "common knowledge" and therefore not a new invention. A patent will be awarded as long as some of the claims are unique as judged by the examiner in the United States patent office. It usually is a worthwhile process to meet with the examiner and make a presentation to distinguish between "prior art" and the current invention. The presentation should focus on those claims that are pivotal that the examiner has judged covered by prior art.

PATENT COOPERATION TREATY APPLICATIONS

The Patent Cooperation Treaty (PCT) is an international agreement for filing applications in many countries abroad. This allows an inventor to file a single international patent application in one language with one patent office while seeking protection in several PCT member countries listed (http://www .uspto.gov/web/offices/pac/dapp/pctstate.html). By January 2010, 147 countries were included in this agreement. In most cases it can be worthwhile to do a PCT application, although there will be additional fees associated with filing particularly in some countries.

LICENSING A PATENT

Once a patent has been filed, the university or the institution may want to grant a license for the patent to a company that agrees to commercialize the invention. Licensing can also be a reiterative process in that some companies involving venture capitalists may invest in the initial development of the invention in order to then grant the license at higher fees to a larger company that has added capital needed to take the invention to market. Licensing fees and the license agreement will have terms on how much the university or institution will receive in royalties and how much investors at each stage along the way will receive. Some portion is also required to be paid to the inventor.

This is an investment decision on the part of the company; when buying a license, they are making a significant decision to invest in the further development of the invention. For a company to invest, they want to be assured that they will have sole use of the invention and restrict competition for 14 years from the time that the patent is awarded (refer to http://www.uspto .gov/inventors/patents.jsp).

Institutional Foundations

Many universities have incorporated separate foundations or companies that can establish companies to further develop their inventions. In this way, the university can maintain its nonprofit status while the commercial development of inventions can be pursued before licensing the patent to a company. By performing further development, they are able to charge higher fees and greater return in royalties from the licensing company. In this way, the university remains nonprofit but can gain further research and development funding as has occurred at the University of Florida at Gainesville.

Medical Inventions

For medical drugs, biologics, and devices, considerable development often is needed to demonstrate safety and efficacy to obtain approval from the Food and Drug Administration to market the invention. This adds greatly to the expense of marketing a drug, device, or biologic as the company usually sponsors the clinical trials before the invention can be marketed in the United States (Figure 11–2). There are recognized phases of clinical trials that a new biologic, drug, or device must pass. Each phase is increasingly expensive and

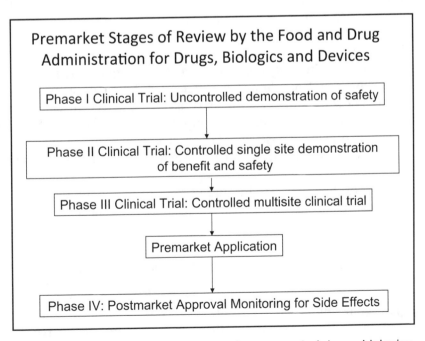

FIGURE 11–2. The premarket stages for approval of drugs, biologics, and devices.

after each phase, the company must decide whether or not the new invention has adequate potential profitability to warrant the additional expense. Decisions about profitability often are the reasons that a new drug or device will not make it to market; only a very small number ever reach the market approval stage with the FDA.

REGULATIONS REGARDING CLINICAL TRIALS

Clinical trials evaluate new treatments (drugs, devices, biologics, and surgical procedures), assess the accuracy of new diagnostic procedures, determine the degree of benefit from preventative procedures, establish the specificity and sensitivity of screening methods, or determine the degree of benefit of altering a patient's quality of life (http://clinicaltrials.gov/ct2/info/understand#Q19).

The first stage is usually a Phase I trial to demonstrate safety of a new medication, device or procedure, the safety of a range of dosages, and the side effects (adverse events) associated with the new treatment. These trials often involve between 20 and 80 patients and likely cost less than later stages of clinical trials.

Phase II clinical trials usually include larger numbers of patients (between 100 and 300), typically include a control group receiving the current standard of care, and are aimed at determining the degree of benefit of the new treatment or diagnostic technique and its side effects or adverse events. These trials can be costly depending on the intervention and the cost of care for the disease or disorder being treated.

Phase III trials are usually large multicenter trials including a control therapy group and involving between 1000 and 3000 patients. The purpose is to determine benefit and monitor side effects at different dosages to demonstrate that the new treatment can be used safely. These trials usually cost several millions of dollars and therefore companies usually do not move to this stage unless the previous Phase I and Phase II trials have shown the new treatment or procedure is safe and has a greater benefit than the current standard of care.

Phase IV are follow-up studies monitoring use after the drug has been cleared for marketing examining side effects, dosages, and safety.

REQUIRED REPORTING OF CLINICAL TRIALS

In the past, companies were not required to report all of the clinical trials conducted on devices, biologics, or drugs, and negative trials often did not get reported or published. Selective reporting meant that often only successful trials were reported but that those not showing benefit or with significant adverse events might not have been divulged. In 1997 the FDA modernization act identified the need for reporting all clinical trials being conducted or sponsored both by government and private industry. In 2002 the FDA developed a "Guidance for Industry Information Program on Clinical Trials for Serious or Life-Threatening Diseases and Conditions" (http://www.fda.gov/downloads/RegulatoryInformation/Guidances/UCM126838.pdf) requiring that all clinical trials sponsored by companies or supported by grants must be registered with http://clinical trials.gov.

In 2007, Public Law 110-85 was issued by the 110th Congress (http://frwebgate.access.gpo.gov/cgi-bin/getdoc.cgi?dbname=110_cong_public_laws&docid=f:publ085.110.pdf, Food and Drug Administration Amendments Act of 2007 or FDAAA), Title VIII, Section 801 requiring that a "responsible party" (that is, either the sponsor or designated principal investigator) register and report results of certain "applicable clinical trials": Applicable trials are prospective controlled, clinical investigations, other than Phase I investigations, of drugs and biologics subject to FDA regulation; and for any controlled trials of devices with health outcomes of a product subject to FDA regulation (other than small feasibility studies), and pediatric postmarket surveillance studies. The Web site http://clinicaltrials.gov was developed by the National Institutes of Health to support reporting of all clinical trials and now hold records of over 85,000 trials from over 170 countries worldwide.

The sponsor or investigator is required to register the trial at the http://clinicaltrials.gov Web site within 21 days of enrolling patients. In addition, there is the requirement that the raw data set or the summary tables must be posted within one year of completion of the trial, that is, when the last patient was discharged. This requirement started in 2009 and 2010 and it is expected that the results will be posted before they are submitted to a journal for publication. Most medical journals now require that a clinical trial is registered with http://clinicaltrials.gov and the data are provided in http://clinicaltrials.gov before the research can be published.

GOOD CLINICAL PRACTICE COMPLIANCE

The FDA Code of Federal Regulations (CFR) Title 21 (http://www.accessdata.fda.gov/scripts/cdrh/cfdocs/cfcfr/CFRSearch.cfm) contains all of the regulations that are legally enforceable laws. That is, an investigator can be prosecuted for not following the regulations in CFR Title 21. In addition, the FDA also provides guidance to investigators on good clinical practices that are in agreement with the European Union International Conference on Harmonization Regulations on the conduct of clinical trials (http://www.ich.org/LOB/media/MEDIA482.pdf).

The CFR Title 21 contains several different sections. For Food and Drugs, Part 11 covers Electronic Records and electronic signatures, Part 50 covers protection of Human Subjects, Part 54 is on Financial Disclosure by Clinical Investigators, Part 56 is on Institutional Review Boards, Part 312 is on Investigation New Drug (IND) Applications, and Part 314 is on Applications for FDA Approval to Market a new Drug. A similar handbook is for the conduct of research on medical devices which contains Parts 11, 50, 54, 56, and Part 807 Establishment Registration and Device Listing for Manufacturers and Initial Importers of Devices, Part 812 on Investigational Device Exemptions, Part 814 Premarket Approval of Medical Devices, Part 820 Quality Systems Regulations, and the 510k and Premarket Approval (PMA) Guidance Document. Each of these can be downloaded from the FDA Web site.

The International Conference on Harmonization (ICH) (http://www.ich .org/cache/compo/276-254-1.html) provides regulations on human research which are not enforceable by the FDA but recommended for guidance. The ICH is accepted by regulatory authorities of Europe, Japan, and the United States. Many documents of the ICH are very specific to conducting trials for certain types of conditions such as cardiac arrhythmias. However, the document on Good Clinical Practice E6(R1) is generic to all types of human research can be downloaded (http://www.ich.org/LOB/media/MEDIA482.pdf) and is highly recommended.

THE ROLES OF THE SPONSOR AND INVESTIGATORS IN FDA-MONITORED CLINICAL TRIALS

The company usually is the sponsor of a trial and responsible for drug or device manufacturing practices and the principal investigator may be a faculty member at a university medical center and is responsible for meeting all of the Title 21 regulations as well as following the ICH Guidelines for Good Clinical Practice. The sponsor reports on the manufacturing quality controls for the drug, biologic, or device directly to the FDA whereas the principal investigator is responsible for writing the application for the research either as an application for an investigational new drug (IND) or an investigational device exemption (IDE). Clinical trial requirements for new drugs are covered by IND and New Drug Applications 21 CFR §312 and §314, for biologics are covered by CFR §312 and §601 and for new devices are covered by Investigational Device Exemptions/5210k/Pre Marketing Application CFR §812 and §814. All of these require IRB Review and Approval, Informed Consent, Form 1572 (for drugs and biologics) and investigator agreement and credentials for devices, and the general investigational plan (for drugs and biologics) and the specific investigational plan for devices.

For drugs, biologics, and devices to be approved for market, there must be substantial evidence based on several controlled investigations to support claims of effectiveness. Applications to conduct a clinical trial of a new drug must be submitted to the FDA as an investigational drug application (IND), whereas device clinical trials are submitted as investigational device exemption (IDE). For both types of applications, a sponsor and a principal investigator are designated.

The FDA conducts routine audits of a portion of clinical trials to verify that the data and procedures are being conducted correctly. FDA examiners will arrive at a site unannounced and ask to review the records demonstrating how the investigational plan is being carried out. The FDA is concerned with evaluating how the data are being collected, validated, and monitored for quality control. They will want to review individual case record forms for patients for completeness and data integrity against the original medical records (source data verification), the standard operating procedures (SOP) guidelines and policies developed, data collection plans, case record form procedures, documentation of staff training, methods and personnel involved in monitoring data collection and recording, and tracking of drugs or devices dispensed.

Depending on the results, they will issue a letter saying either that the research is in full compliance with CFR Title 21, that the investigators have some objectionable practices that are not major departures from regulations, or a warning letter where investigators' practices are significant departures from regulations. If a clinical investigator has repeated FDA instances of violations of regulations, they will be disqualified from overseeing further investigations. There is public disclosure of disqualified investigators by the FDA on the Internet.

DEFINING THE ROLES OF PERSONS INVOLVED THE CLINICAL TRIALS

The principal investigator (PI) is responsible for following all of the regulations contained in the CFR Title 21 of the FDA and following good clinical practice guidelines of the International Conference on Harmonization (ICH E6 Guideline Consolidated Document on Good Clinical Practice). Investigators for drug studies must sign FDA Form 1572 (http://www.fda.gov/downloads/AboutFDA/ReportsManualsForms/Forms/UCM074728.pdf) providing information on their qualifications and their agreement to follow 21 CFR part 312 regulations. Of particular concern are 312.64 on investigators reports, 312.50 on obtaining informed consent, 312.54 on informing investigators, 312.62 on investigator recordkeeping and record retention, and 312.68 on inspection of investigator's records and reports. Therefore, as the PI is responsible for maintaining compliance with all aspects of CFR Title 312 and following the guidance of the ICH, they must be familiar with all of these regulations as well as being qualified in the area under investigation (Figure 11-3). For this reason, their CV must also be submitted to the FDA with Form 1572.

Many medical schools now offer masters degrees in clinical investigation for physicians planning to become PIs on clinical trials. These are listed on the Web page of the Association of American Medical Colleges (http://www.aamc

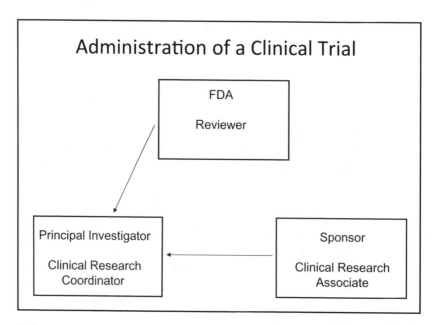

FIGURE 11–3. The relationship of the principal investigator with the sponsor and the FDA.

.org/research/clinicalresearch/training/start.htm). Currently about 62 medical colleges offer these programs for physicians.

The sponsor usually is the company responsible for the manufacturing of the drug, device or biologic. The PI and the sponsors are independent to reduce conflict of interest; that is, if the PI is an employee of the company they may be under pressure from the sponsor to make certain the results are efficacious. Thus, it is important to show that the PI does not own stock in the company or is receiving payment contingent on the results of the research.

The PI usually hires a clinical research coordinator (CRC) who works under their direction to perform many of the tasks for record keeping, coordination, and data validation. Such persons are often nurse practitioners who have received additional training on the conduct of clinical trials. Some have taken master's degrees in clinical investigation along with physicians. These courses provide backgrounds in epidemiology, biostatistics, FDA regulations, the roles of the IRB, and the ICH Guidelines on good clinical practices. The role of the CRC is paramount as the PI usually is a medical faculty member with heavy teaching and patient care responsibilities in addition to being a clinical investigator. Others who may serve as CRCs are registered medical assistants who are certified and trained in programs accredited by two agencies, the Commission on Accreditation of Allied Health Education Programs (CAAHEP) and the Accreditation Bureau of Health Education Schools (ABHES).

A third person involved in monitoring the research is a clinical research associate (CRA) who monitors the conduct of the research on behalf of the company sponsoring the research to ensure that all FDA regulations are being followed correctly and that adequate data verification procedures are met. The CRA may visit the coordinating site for a multicenter trial on a frequent basis—once every 6 weeks or so. Their responsibility is to ensure that the investigator follows the investigational plan, that the team enters the data correctly and accurately, that they follow FDA regulations, and comply with the procedures established by the sponsor.

PUBLICATION OF THE RESULTS OF CLINICAL TRIALS

Usually, the sponsor has a contract with the medical school or university of the principal investigator. Independence of the PI must be ensured, particularly when it comes to publication. Often, the company will have preview rights provided for in the contract that allows the sponsor to review the data and the manuscript for a 30-day period before submission for publication or before presentation at a scientific meeting. However, although the company may make suggestions after the prereview, care must be taken in the terms of the agreement to ensure that the PI does not need to change the manuscript based on input from the company. Also, the agreement must recognize the need for the PI and the PI's staff to maintain independence and that the peer-review process must not be interfered with leading to publication of the results. As mentioned earlier, most medical journals now require that the data set be provided (to http://www.clincialtrials.gov) prior to submission for publication.

Financial disclose of conflicts of interest are required when an article is published, which must include information on who provided financial support for the study, what was supported by the sponsor, and whether or not the principal investigator has any personal holdings in the company.

12

Wrapping It Up

As we noted earlier in this book, the successful scientist has expertise in at least one field of study but also masters skills and capabilities that go beyond knowledge of a scientific specialty. One of our main goals is to identify and describe information and resources that pertain to the various facets of a career in research, including career planning, designing and managing a research program, writing and publishing, submitting research grant applications, succeeding in academia, and obtaining patents. Much of the information is universal in its application—it applies broadly to several disciplines in the biomedical sciences, medical/surgical careers in clinical research, physical sciences, and the allied health sciences. Inevitably, discipline-specific issues need to be considered, but broad strokes are sufficient to paint the landscape in which scientific careers are formed.

We have tried to be honest in our appraisal. Certainly, we are eager to proclaim the satisfactions of a career in science, but we do not want to neglect or minimize the difficult challenges, occasional frustrations, and downright failures that are part of science. Our experience, like that of a host of scientists, is that the rewards of a scientific career far outweigh the disadvantages. There is a privilege in being a scientist and that privilege is earned through education and effort.

We now offer summary advice on some of the building blocks in a scientific career. This advice is given in the spirit of suggestions for you to consider. We do not pretend that every suggestion will work for every person in every circumstance. Some of these points are refinements and elaborations of points made in earlier chapters.

INTERVIEWING SKILLS

Even highly educated and experienced individuals sometimes fail to interview effectively. Interviewing for positions is an opportunity to showcase individual abilities and potential, as well as to explore the circumstances of employment. Some scientists are inappropriately taciturn because they are reluctant to "blow their own horn"; others talk incessantly during an interview and leave few opportunities for the interviewer to break in with necessary questions. Interviewing is an art, both for the one giving the interview and for the one being interviewed. In a job interview, the applicant should try to learn about the company, agency, or institution and department that is offering employment. This means becoming familiar with its products, services, or specialties. Searches on the Internet are a good first step. It can be helpful to learn as many names of current employees (especially those on the interview schedule) and their credentials before the interview. It can be difficult to learn many names as possible during the interview itself, and most people like to be recognized by their names. Likewise, prospective employees generally are pleased when an applicant has taken steps to know more about them.

Although this chapter cannot offer detailed advice on every kind of interview, we suggest a few general pointers:

1. *Be candid and honest.* It is fine to say, "I don't know" if you are asked about something you are not prepared to discuss. No one knows everything. Admitting ignorance is better than risking an error-filled reply. However, you should feel comfortable in hypothesizing or speculating, as long as you make it clear that is what you are doing.

2. *Make your answers concise and informative.* Don't feel the need to keep talking once you have made your central point. Interviews are not lectures or monologues. Most interviewers come prepared with a set of questions that need to be answered and they can become frustrated if they cannot accomplish their objectives because the person being interviewed talks incessantly.

3. *Be courteous.* Attend carefully to the questions you are asked and be sure you understand them before you answer. If you are unclear about a question, politely ask for a clarification. It is OK to ask, "Did I answer your question?" because it shows that you are sincere.

4. *Be cordial.* You are being sought as a person, not a machine or software program. Interviewers ask themselves, "Would we like working with this person?"

5. *Be prepared to summarize your interests and goals, and to describe how your experiences and skills relate to the job description (very important).* Keep in mind that the prospective employer needs to know

how you will fit in and what you can contribute. If you meet with several people in succession, as is often the case for academic positions, try to articulate a consistent message and to emphasize why you are suited to the position.

6. *Try to have at least one or two questions to ask during your interview.* Asking questions shows that you are interested in the position. But if your interview is a series of interviews with individuals or small groups, don't ask the same question in every individual interview. Such repetition sends a bad message.

7. *Some interviewers will ask questions such as "What is your primary strength?" or "What is your primary weakness?" or "What have you found to most difficult in your previous jobs?"* It helps to think about these kinds of questions before the interview. Increasingly popular are behavior-based questions, on the assumption that your previous experiences are a good indication of how you will respond to problems and challenges in the future. For example, an interview question might be: (1) "Describe a time when you observed a coworker or supervisor make a serious error. How did you respond, and what did you learn from this experience?" (2) "If you have supervised lab staff, how did you encourage them to work diligently and accurately?" (3) "Describe an experience in which you needed to acquire a new skill to perform your job. How did you go about it?" Although it is not possible to predict exactly what questions may be asked at a particular interview, it can help to practice answering questions of this kind.

8. *Give thought before the interview to conditions of employment.* For example, an applicant for an academic position should be able to outline their intended research program for the first 5 years and provide a start-up package (for laboratory equipment, laboratory staff, and supplies) for meeting the plan along with expectations regarding reduction in courses to be taught. Usually, it is sufficient to "ballpark" the start-up package and define it more thoroughly as negotiations warrant. An exorbitant request for a start-up may bring things to a quick and final termination. Depending on the employing organization, it may be appropriate to mention your salary requirements. When interviewing for academic appointments, it usually is possible to learn salary ranges from public sources. It is not a good idea to dwell on items such as vacation allowance or sick leave, because it sends a bad message. It is your enthusiasm for the work, along with your qualifications, that makes you attractive to a potential employer.

9. *Bring extra copies of your resume or abbreviated CV* (see next section). Some applicants offer a copy as they sit down to begin the interview. Interviewers can use this copy to refresh their memories, make personal notes, or highlight sections of special interest. It can be appropriate to make selective reference to items in your resume or CV during the interview.

This can help the interviewer to identify key aspects of your experience or knowledge.

10. *After the interview, follow up with a note expressing your gratitude for the interview opportunity.* It can be appropriate to include a brief comment on your enthusiasm for the job in question. If warranted, it is also an opportunity to follow up on items raised during the interview, such as additional information on lab equipment needed for startup to the Chair of the Search Committee.

TAILORED RESUMES

Many scientists acquire a variety of skills and types of knowledge. Some may be more relevant than others when applying for a particular job, research grant, fellowship, or other opportunity. Therefore, preparation of resumes tailored to specific opportunities can be a positive step. Scientists who are early in their careers may not need anything beyond a single resume or CV, but more experienced scientists, especially those who have worked in a variety of areas, are well-advised to craft resumes that reflect their expertise and experience in relevant specialties. Preparing resumes of different length and for different purposes also is worthwhile. For example, a scientist may prepare an NIH biosketch (Chapter 7), a comprehensive CV (Chapters 8 and 10), an abridged CV (sometimes requested for purposes that do not call for a full CV (e.g., to document expertise in writing letters of recommendation, providing credentials for consulting), and biosketches of 100 or 250 words (often used in brief blurbs for programs at scientific meetings, announcements of various kinds, and brochures). Take care in preparing resumes and CVs. Both content and style matter. A well-constructed resume or CV attracts favorable attention and helps to remind others of your skills and experiences. It is surprising how many resumes and CVs contain mistakes, inconsistencies, and misleading information. After you have completed a CV or resume, ask yourself if it represents you in the way you want to be represented. Then ask a colleague to review it as though he or she were a prospective employer. Of course, it is good practice to update resumes and CVs at regular intervals, and to add categories of professional accomplishment as appropriate. Categories delineate particular experiences and skills that change over time.

JOB TALKS

Whether one is applying for a first position or a job change, the interview usually requires a job talk. This is an opportunity to demonstrate expertise in a subject area, to point to promising areas of future work, and perhaps to outline a research program. An immediate question to consider is: who is your audience? If your audience is peer scientists, then you can assume a good deal of shared knowledge. But if your audience consists in part of individuals who are not well acquainted with your specialty, then be prepared to define terms and explain concepts that would be familiar to specialists.

We strongly recommend practicing a job talk, even if your audience is only a few obliging friends. Video-recording your talk is a good practice and can be highly revealing of strengths and weaknesses. Some go a step further and ask for professional assessments of their presentation skills. Whatever your audience, ask for candid assessments about organization of the talk, presentation style, clarity and value of illustrations, and so on. The objective is to get honest and constructive criticism, so you might go so far as to prepare an evaluation form that pointedly asks the audience member to rate and comment on various aspects of your talk. Practicing the talk helps you to accomplish a smooth flow of ideas and to work out matters of timing. All too often, speakers have too much content for the time available and try to rush though the final information in an effort to get it all in. As a consequence, the talk seems poorly organized, the final points are blurred, and both the speaker and the audience feel frazzled.

Carefully review your visual aids. Examine your slides to check for clarity and accuracy. Avoid slides that challenge the viewer with information overload or information that is difficult to see from a distance. Try to make smooth transitions between slides, for example, by explaining, "This point is further developed in the next slide" or "We realized that an additional control [or analysis] was needed to confirm our findings." Keep to the time limit given for your talk. If time is allotted for questions and discussion, be sure to accommodate it. While giving the talk, scan the audience to make occasional eye contact in different parts of the room. It can be disconcerting to the audience when a speaker avoids eye contact or makes such contact with only a fraction of the audience. Tasteful humor helps to make the audience comfortable, but jokes should not stand in the way of a serious scientific message.

A Little Help from Friends and Supporters

Finding employment, getting promoted, and receiving grants and awards often hinge on letters of recommendation. Every scientist should have a list of individuals who can submit letters of recommendation. It can facilitate things to keep these individuals informed of career changes, new projects, recently acquired skills, accomplishments, and career goals. A letter writer who is so informed can emphasize points that are especially relevant. Certainly, it helps to send letter writers not only an updated resume or CV, but a succinct summary of one's current situation and plans for the future can provide a perspective that is often lacking or inexplicit in a resume.

Do what you can to make the task of a letter writer easy and straightforward. Sending a 30-page CV requires the writer to scan through a great deal of information to identify the most relevant pieces. It is highly recommended that you ask permission from potential letter writers to mention their names to a prospective employer beforehand. If they consent, then it is appropriate to send them background information for the position, unless the prospective employer assumes the responsibility of contacting them. Letters of recommendation vary from those that are "damning with faint praise" to others that are substantive and highly supportive. Although it usually is not a good idea to exercise much influence on what a letter writer actually says, it is appropriate to express concisely your qualifications for a position and to describe how the position relates to your career goals. It can be a great assistance to letter writers if they know why you believe you are highly qualified for a particular position.

STARTING WELL, FINISHING WELL

A first job can open future opportunities but also restrict them. This might sound a bit elitist, but here is the advice we have heard from some of our colleagues in academia. Taking a first job in a university that does not have a strong national reputation can have the effect of limiting future employment in universities that are highly regarded. It is not simply a matter of institutional reputation but also a matter of resources, of colleagues, and of opportunities. "Moving up" from one institutional tier to another is by no means impossible, but it can be difficult. We know of circumstances in which deans or other administrators disregarded job candidates because their current position was with an institution considered to be of lower tier. Certainly, there can be good reasons to begin a career with an institution or department that does not enjoy the highest reputation, so this point of advice has to be evaluated against individual circumstances.

LAB MISSION STATEMENT

Lab mission statements were mentioned in Chapter 9. These are worthwhile for many reasons. They can be succinct statements of a lab's research goals, philosophy, and ways of operating. Such statements can be valuable touchstones for newly hired personnel, students in training, lab visitors, or anyone interested in the research accomplished at the lab. Lab mission statements generally summarize the main research goals (e.g., to understand the genetic bases of a particular form of cancer), but they can extend to standards of laboratory practice, expectations of lab personnel, and schedules of lab meetings. Some are crafted to provide elaborated information about a lab; a good example is the mission statement of the Special Pathogens Branch of the Centers for Disease Control (http://www.cdc.gov/ncidod/dvrd/spb/mnpages/whoweare.htm). Other mission statements are briefer, outlining three or four major goals or objectives. Mission statements vary with the type of work done in the laboratory and the purpose to be accomplished. They do not take the place of a manual of standard operating procedures (Chapter 6) but are useful for general orientation and description of a lab's purpose.

FIVE-YEAR PLANS

Many organizations ask their employees to prepare long-term plans, and some individuals formulate such plans for their own benefit even if there is no mandate for their preparation. There is nothing magic about any particular period of projection, but 5 years is typical for long-term planning in science. It is long enough to think about a career trajectory but short enough to be realistic and to anticipate opportunities and challenges. It is also a reasonable period of time for major accomplishments, which is why many federal research grants have 5 years of project duration.

KEEP GROWING

To be current, a scientist must respond to advances in knowledge and technology, changes in work environment, need for new skills, and challenges of job promotion or job changes. Some of the changes can be anticipated or planned, others will simply happen because of external circumstances. Although the future cannot be predicted with certainty, it often is possible to identify knowledge or skills that are highly likely to improve job performance or lead to promotions. Once these are identified, the next step is to plan for how and when they will be acquired.

PUBLISH HIGH-QUALITY RESEARCH IN HIGH IMPACT JOURNALS

Regardless of all other factors, building a high quality productive publication record is the ticket to developing research credentials and a solid reputation as a scientist. Your reputation will depend on your publication record in high impact peer-reviewed journals and is essential to opening the doors to all aspects of success in science such as promotion and tenure, new opportunities, grant funding, institutional support, and awards. Above all else, taking care to develop a high-quality research publication record should be a major focus, particularly early in your career. Some of the following tips are provided as publishing hints.

1. Review journals carefully before submitting your work. Select a journal that has a high impact and is broad in scope, but appropriate for your work.

2. Write your article with the journal in mind. Most high-impact journals have a broad mission and therefore the article has to be written knowing that some of the reviewers may not have expertise in your specialty.

3. Always write a letter to the Editor on why your work is significant and well matched to the mission/scope of the journal. Sometimes submitting an abstract to the Editor can save you time as it allows the Editor to let you know whether your article is of interest or not. It is essential that you let the Editor know why the work is of significance and well matched to the mission of the journal. Review the mission/scope of the journal and address that in your letter.

4. When you receive a request for revision, attend to each point and take care to address it directly. You may express disagreement but when a revision ignores some of the reviewer's advice, it can cause a very negative reaction. Reviewers are voluntarily taking the time to do reviews and expect to have a proper response to their concerns.

5. When you receive a rejection, look at the reasons carefully. If the reviewers found a fatal flaw in the study, consider redoing the study appropriately rather than risk your reputation by publishing poor quality science. One published poor quality study can come back to haunt you later if a grant reviewer happened to read it and remember you as publishing poor quality research.

6. If the article was rejected because of its limited scope for a high-impact journal, then revising the article to address the concerns of the reviewers and then submitting to a more appropriate journal is essential. If the research is of adequate quality to be published, then revising the article and submitting after rejection is necessary. Wise authors have used reviewers' comments to improve their manuscripts before submitting them to another journal.

7. Take care if an article is rejected for scientific quality reasons by journals, perhaps it should not be published as doing so might reflect badly on you and your co-authors.

8. Focus early in your career on publishing original research in peer-reviewed journals, Chapters in books and books should only be considered later in a career and should always be fewer in number than peer-reviewed research articles.

Scientists should always keep in mind that their publication record is their reputation and make that their primary focus particularly for the first decade of their career as it will directly impact their resources and funding. Also, their publication record determines whether they will be sought out by high-quality postdoctoral candidates and are able to obtain research grants.

MAINTAINING A PROFESSIONAL RELATIONSHIP WITH YOUR PEERS

Finally, remembering that you are part of a community of scientists is important. Always maintain a respectful relationship with others even when you disagree with them on scientific issues. When a scientific disagreement becomes public, both members of the disagreement can be harmed. Although a lively discussion at scientific meetings is excellent and useful, it should never become personal. Disagreeing with a colleague should be possible without interfering with a cordial relationship. However, at the same time, be aware than not everyone is capable of such behavior. When selecting referees to recommend for reviewers of an article, you are submitting to a journal always be careful not to list persons who might disagree with your line of research. However, when possible, you should select leaders in the field; this is one way for them to become aware of your research.

CONCLUSION

Building a research career is not something that simply happens. We hope that we have given the reader the knowledge of the necessary tools, methods, and guidance needed to navigate the process. Although science is demanding as a career, it also is unparalleled in the amount of excitement and satisfaction that can be reaped. Although not a 9 to 5 job, but one that requires discipline, hard work, and imagination, it can be highly rewarding in a personnel sense as well as providing the support and friendship of others from around the world. We hope this book will help others to enjoy the immense rewards of a research career.

References

Aickin, M., & Gensler, H. (1996). Adjusting for multiple testing when reporting research results: The Bonferroni vs. Holm methods. *American Journal of Public Health, 86*(5), 726–728.

American Psychological Association. (2001). *Publication manual of the American Psychological Association* (5th ed.). Washington, DC: APA Books.

Ashburner, J., & Friston, K. J. (2000). Voxel-based morphometry—the methods. *Neuroimage, 11*(6, Pt. 1), 805–821.

Atlas, M. C. (2003). Emerging ethical issues in instructions to authors of high-impact biomedical journals. *Journal of the Medical Librarians Association, 91*(4), 442–449.

Aydingoz, U. (2005). Figures, tables, and references: Integral but sometimes neglected components of scientific articles. *Diagnostic and Interventional Radiology, 11*(2), 67–68.

Bekelman, J. E., Li, Y., & Gross, C. P. (2003). Scope and impact of financial conflicts of interest in biomedical research: A systematic review. *Journal of the Amerian Medical Association, 289*(4), 454–465.

Benos, D. J., Bashari, E., Chaves, J. M., Gaggar, A., Kapoor, N., LaFrance, M., . . . Zotov, A. (2007). The ups and downs of peer review. *Advances in Physiology Education, 31*(2), 145–152.

Benos, D. J., Fabres, J., Farmer, J., Gutierrez, J. P., Hennessy, K., Kosek, D., et al. (2005). Ethics and scientific publication. *Advances in Physiology Education, 29*(2), 59–74.

Berberet, H. (2008, June). Perceptions of early career faculty: Managing the transition from graduate school to the professional career. New York, NY: TIAA-CREF Institute: Research Dialog.

Berk, R. A. (2006). *Thirteen strategies to meaure college teaching.* Sterling, VA: Stylus.

Bonetta, L. E. (2006). *Making the right moves: A practical guide to scientific management for postdocs and new faculty* (2nd ed.). Research Triangle, NC: Burrough Wellcome Fund and Chevy Chase, MD: Howard Hughes Medical Institute.

Bossuyt, P. M., Reitsma, J. B., Bruns, D. E., Gatsonis, C. A., Glasziou, P. P., Irwig, L. M., . . . Lijmer, J. (2003). The STARD statement for reporting studies of diagnostic accuracy: Explanation and elaboration. *Annals of Internal Medicine, 138*(1), W1–W12.

Boullata, J. I., & Mancuso, C. E. (2007). A "how-to" guide in preparing abstracts and poster presentations. *Nutrition in Clinical Practice, 22*(6), 641–646.

Boutron, I., Moher, D., Altman, D. G., Schulz, K. F., & Ravaud, P. (2008). Extending the CONSORT statement to randomized trials of nonpharmacologic treatment: Explanation and elaboration. *Annals of Internal Medicine, 148*(4), 295–309.

Brumback, R. A. (2009). Success at publishing in biomedical journals: Hints from a journal editor. *Journal of Child Neurology, 24*(3), 370–378.

Butler, D. (2005). Electronic notebooks: A new leaf. *Nature, 436*(7047), 20–21.

Cancer Therapy Evaluation Program. (1999). Common toxicity criteria manual, Version 2.0 and Common toxicity criteria (CTC).

Carmichael, H. L. (1988).Incentives in academics: why is there tenure?" *Journal of Political Economy*, 96, 453–472.

Chargaff, E. (1976). Triviality in science: A brief meditation on fashions. *Perspectives in Biology and Medicine, 19*, 324–333.

Charlton, B. G. (2006). Scientific life should be measured in seven year units [Editorial]. *Medical Hypotheses*, 66, 1051–1052.

Charmaz, K. (2006). *Constructing grounded theory.* Thousand Oaks, CA: Sage Publications.

Chelvarajah, R., & Bycroft, J. (2004). Writing and publishing case reports: The road to success. *Acta Neurochirurgica (Wien), 146*(3), 313–316; discussion 316.

Chen, C., Hu, Q., Yan, J., Yang, X., Shi, X., Lei, J., . . . Zhou, C. (2009). Early inhibition of HIF-1alpha with small interfering RNA reduces ischemic-reperfused brain injury in rats. *Neurobiology of Disease, 33*(3), 509–517.

Chen, C. C., Brucke, C., Kempf, F., Kupsch, A., Lu, C. S., Lee, S. T., . . . Brown, P. (2006). Deep brain stimulation of the subthalamic nucleus: A two-edged sword. *Current Biology, 16*(22), R952–R953.

Claxton, L. D. (2005). Scientific authorship. Part 2. History, recurring issues, practices, and guidelines. *Mutant Research, 589*(1), 31–45.

Cohen, J. (1992). A power primer. *Psychological Bulletin, 112*(1), 155–159.

Correia, A. S., Anisimov, S. V., Li, J. Y., & Brundin, P. (2005). Stem cell-based therapy for Parkinson's disease. *Annals of Medicine, 37*(7), 487–498.

Coscarelli, S., Verrecchia, L., Le Saec, O., Coscarelli, A., Santoro, R., & de Campora, E. (2007). Rehabilitation protocol of dysphagia after subtotal reconstructive laryngectomy. *Acta Otorhinolaryngolica Italica, 27*(6), 286–289.

Council of Biology Editors. (1968). Proposed definition of a primary publication. *Newsletter, Council of Biology Editors*, November 1969, pp. 1–2.; as cited by: Day, Robert A. (1994). *How to write and publish a scientific paper.* Phoenix, AZ: Oryx Press, p. 9.

Creswell, J. (1998). *Qualitative inquiry and research design: Choosing among the five traditions.* Thousand Oaks, CA: Sage Publications.

Creswell, J., & Plano Clark, V. L. (2007). *Designing and conducting mixed methods research.* Thousand Oaks, CA: Sage Publications.

Damp, D. V. (2008). *The book of U.S. government jobs* (10th ed.). Mckees Rocks, PA: Bookhaven.

Davis, G. (2005). Doctors without orders. *American Scientist, 93*(Suppl. 3). Available from: http://postdoc.sigmaxi.org/results/.

Des Jarlais, D. C., Lyles, C., & Crepaz, N. (2004). Improving the reporting quality of nonrandomized evaluations of behavioral and public health interventions: The TREND statement. *American Journal of Public Health, 94*(3), 361–366.

Deuschl, G., Schade-Brittinger, C., Krack, P., Volkmann, J., Schafer, H., Botzel, K., et al. (2006). A randomized trial of deep-brain stimulation for Parkinson's disease. *New England Journal of Medicine, 355*(9), 896–908.

Doyle, H., Gass, A., & Kennison, R. (2004a). Open access and scientific societies. *PLoS Biology, 2*(5), E156.

Doyle, H., Gass, A., & Kennison, R. (2004b). Who pays for open access? *PLoS Biology, 2*(4), E105.

Editors, I. C. o. M. J. (2008, October). *Uniform requirements for manuscritps submitted to biomedical journals: Writing and editing for biomedical publication.* Available from: http://www.icmje.org.

Emanuel, E. J., Wendler, D., & Grady, C. (2000). What makes clinical research ethical? *Journal of the American Medical Association, 283*(31), 2701–2711.

Ethics, C.-C. o. P. (1999). *Guidelines on good publication practice.* Available from: http://www.publicationethics.org.uk.

Eysenbach, G., & Kummervold, P. E. (2005). "Is cybermedicine killing you?"—The story of a Cochrane disaster. *Journal of Medical Internet Research, 7*(2), e21.

Food and Drug Administration. (1995). *Guideline for industry: Clinical safety data management: Definitions and standards for expedited reporting.* Retrieved May 21, 2010, from http://www.fda.gov/downloads/Drugs/GuidanceComplianceRegulatoryInformation/Guidances/ucm073087.pdfFood and Drug Administration. (1999). International Conference on Harmonisation: Choice of control group in clinical trials. *Federal Register, 64,* 51767–51780.

Francis, C. K. (2001). The medical ethos and social responsibility in clinical medicine. *Journal of the National Medical Association, 93,* 157–169.

Friedman, L., & Richter, E. D. (2005). Conflicts of interest and scientific integrity. *International Journal of Occupational and Environmental Health, 11*(2), 205–206.

Friedman, P. J. (1990). Correcting the literature following fraudulent publication. *Journal of the American Medical Association, 263*(10), 1416–1419.

Garcia, A. M. (2004). Sixth version of the "Uniform Requirements for Manuscripts Submitted to Biomedical Journals": Lots of ethics, some new recommendations for manuscript preparation. *Journal of Epidemiology and Community Health, 58*(9), 731–733.

Glänzel, W. (2006). On the opportunities and limitations of the H-index. *Science Focus, 1,* 10–11.

Gliner, J. A., Morgan, G. A., & Harmon, R. J. (2002a). The chi-square test and accompanying effect size indices. *Journal of the American Academy of Child and Adolescent Psychiatry, 41*(12), 1510–1512.

Gliner, J. A., Morgan, G. A., & Harmon, R. J. (2002b). Single-factor repeated-measures designs: Analysis and interpretation. *Journal of the American Academy of Child and Adolescent Psychiatry, 41*(8), 1014–1016.

Gliner, J. A., Morgan, G. A., Leech, N. L., & Harmon, R. J. (2001). Problems with null hypothesis significance testing. *Journal of the American Academy of Child and Adolescent Psychiatry, 40*(2), 250–252.

Goldbort, R. (1998). Scientific writing: Three neglected aspects. *Journal of Environmental Health, 60,* 26–29.

Hames, I. (2008). Digital images and the problems of inappropriate manipulation: Can you believe what you see? *Journal of European Medical Writers Association, 17,* 164–167.

Holm, S. A. (1979). A simple sequentially rejective multiple test procedures. *Scandinavian Journal of Statistics, 6*, 65-70.

Horng, S. H., & Miller, F. G. (2007). Placebo-controlled procedural trials for neurological conditions. *Neurotherapeutics, 4*(3), 531-536.

Imel, Z. E., Wampold, B. E., Miller, S. D., & Fleming, R. R. (2008). Distinctions without a difference: Direct comparisons of psychotherapies for alcohol use disorders. *Psychology of Addictuve Behaviors, 22*(4), 533-543.

International Conference on Harmonisation. (1997). International Conference on Harmonisation of Technical Requirements for Registration of Pharmaceuticals for Human Use (ICH). Good clinical practice, consolidated guidance. *62, Federal Register, 25692*. Available from: http://www.cc.nih.gov/ccc/clinicalresearch/guidance.pdf.

Jacobs, A., Carpenter, J., Donnelly, J., Klapproth, J. F., Gertel, A., Hall, G., et al. (2005). The involvement of professional medical writers in medical publications: Results of a Delphi study. *Current Medical Research and Opinion, 21*(2), 311-316.

Jarvis, E. D. (2004). Learned birdsong and the neurobiology of human language. *Annals of the New York Academy of Sciences, 1016*, 749-777.

Jones, B. F., Wuchty, S., & Uzzi, B. (2008). Multi-university research teams: Shifting impact, geography, and stratification in science. *Science, 322*(5905), 1259-1262.

Jones, M., Gebski, V., Onslow, M., & Packman, A. (2002). Statistical power in stuttering research: A tutorial. *Journal of Speech, Language and Hearing Research, 45*(2), 243-255.

Kariv, Y., Wang, W., Senagore, A. J., Hammel, J. P., Fazio, V. W., & Delaney, C. P. (2006). Multivariable analysis of factors associated with hospital readmission after intestinal surgery. *American Journal of Surgery, 191*(3), 364-371.

Khan, N. L., Jain, S., Lynch, J. M., Pavese, N., Abou-Sleiman, P., Holton, J. L., et al. (2005). Mutations in the gene LRRK2 encoding dardarin (PARK8) cause familial Parkinson's disease: Clinical, pathological, olfactory and functional imaging and genetic data. *Brain, 128*(Pt. 12), 2786-2796.

Kliewer, M. A. (2005). Writing it up: A step-by-step guide to publication for beginning investigators. *American Journal of Roentgenology, 185*, 591-596.

Korenman, S., Berk, R. W., Wenger, N. S., & Lew, V. (1998). Evaluation of the research norms of scientists and administrators responsible for academic research integrity. *Journal of the American Medical Association, 279*(1), 41-47.

Kostoff, R. N., & Hartley, J. (2001). Structured abstracts for technical journals. *Science, 292*(5519), 1067.

Kotzin, S., & Schuyler, P. L. (1989). NLM's practices for handling errata and retractions. *Bulletin of the Medical Library Association, 77*(4), 337-342.

Kruger, G. M., & Morrison, S. J. (2002). Brain repair by endogenous progenitors. *Cell, 110*(4), 399-402.

LaMonte, B. H., Wallace, K. E., Holloway, B. A., Shelly, S. S., Ascano, J., Tokito, M., . . . Holzbaur, E. L. (2002). Disruption of dynein/dynactin inhibits axonal transport in motor neurons causing late-onset progressive degeneration. *Neuron, 34*(5), 715-727.

Lang, D. B. (2001). The art of scientific writing. *Radiology, 218*(1), 7.

Lazer, R. (2004). Up for grabs—Authors are a dime a dozen: The problem of multiple authors. *Acta Pediatrica, 93*, 589-591.

Levin, B. (1996). Annotation: On the Holm, Simnes, and Hochberg multiple test procedures. *American Journal of Public Health*, *86*(5), 628-629.

Lichtenwalner, R. J., & Parent, J. M. (2006). Adult neurogenesis and the ischemic forebrain. *Journal of Cerebral Blood Flow and Metabolism*, *26*(1), 1-20.

Martin, B. (1992). Scientific fraud and the power structure of science. *Prometheus*, *10*, 83-98.

Martinson, B. C., Anderson, M. S., & de Vries, R. (2005). Scientists behaving badly. *Nature*, *435*(7043), 737-738.

Mathisen, P. M. (2003). Gene discovery and validation for neurodegenerative diseases. *Drug Discovery Today*, *8*(1), 39-46.

McCarthy, L. H., & Reilly, K. E. (2000). How to write a case report. *Family Medicine*, *32*(3), 190-195.

Medawar, P. B. (1990). Is the scientific paper a fraud? In D. Pyke (Ed.), *The threat and the glory: Reflections on science and scientists*. Oxford, UK: Oxford University Press.

Miller, G. A. (1977). *Spontaneous apprentices: Children and language*. New York, NY: Seabury Press.

Moher, D., Cook, D. J., Eastwood, S., Olkin, I., Rennie, D., & Stroup, D. F. (1999). Improving the quality of reports of meta-analyses of randomised controlled trials: The QUOROM statement. Quality of reporting of meta-analyses. *Lancet*, *354*(9193), 1896-1900.

Moher, D., Schulz, K. F., & Altman, D. (2001). The CONSORT statement: Revised recommendations for improving the quality of reports of parallel-group randomized trials. *Journal of the American Medical Association*, *285*(15), 1987-1991.

Nakatomi, H., Kuriu, T., Okabe, S., Yamamoto, S., Hatano, O., Kawahara, N., . . . Nakafuku, M. (2002). Regeneration of hippocampal pyramidal neurons after ischemic brain injury by recruitment of endogenous neural progenitors. *Cell*, *110*(4), 429-441.

Neely, J. G., Hartman, J. M., Forsen, J. W., Jr., & Wallace, M. S. (2003). Tutorials in clinical research: part VII. Understanding comparative statistics (contrast)—part A: General concepts of statistical significance. *Laryngoscope*, *113*(9), 1534-1540.

Office of Research Integrity. (2001). *Guidelines for assessing possible research misconduct in clinical research and clinical trials*. Retrieved May 21, 2010, from http://ori.dhhs.gov/misconduct/inquiry_issues.shtml

Patel, U. A., Patadia, M. O., Holloway, N., & Rosen, F. (2009). Poor radiotherapy compliance predicts persistent regional disease in advanced head/neck cancer. *Laryngoscope*, *119*(3), 528-533.

Ranstam, J., Buyse, M., George, S. L., Evans, S., Geller, N. L., Scherrer, B., . . . Lachenbruch, P. (2000). Fraud in medical research: An international survey of biostatisticians. ISCB Subcommittee on Fraud. *Controlled Clinical Trials*, *21*(5), 415-427.

Rossner, M., & Yamada, K. M. (2004). What's in a picture? The temptation of image manipulation. *Journal of Cell Biology*, *166*(1), 11-15.

Russell, S. W., & Morrison, D. C. (2010). *The grant application writer's workbook*. Los Olivos, CA: Grant Writers' Seminars and Workshops, LLC.

Schicatano, E. J., Peshori, K. R., Gopalaswamy, R., Sahay, E., & Evinger, C. (2000). Reflex excitability regulates prepulse inhibition. *Journal of Neuroscience*, *20*(11), 4240-4247.

Schriger, D. L., & Cooper, R. J. (2001). Achieving graphical excellence: Suggestions and methods for creating high-quality visual displays of experimental data. *Annals of Emergency Medicine, 37*(1), 75–87.

Schroter, S. (2006). Importance of free access to research articles on decision to submit to the BMJ: Survey of authors. *British Medical Journal, 332*(7538), 394–396.

Schroter, S., & Tite, L. (2006). Open access publishing and author-pays business models: A survey of authors' knowledge and perceptions. *Journal of the Royal Society of Medicine, 99*(3), 141–148.

Schwartzkroin, P. A. (2009). *So you want to be a scientist?* New York, NY: Oxford University Press.

Silverman, F. H. (1988). The "monster" study. *Journal of Fluency Disorders, 13*, 225–231.

Siwek, J., Gourlay, M. L., Slawson, D. C., & Shaughnessy, A. F. (2002). How to write an evidence-based clinical review article. *American Family Physician, 65*(2), 251–258.

Smith, R. (2006). The trouble with medical journals. *Journal of the Royal Society of Medicine, 99*(3), 115–119.

Sollaci, L. B., & Pereira, M. G. (2004). The introduction, methods, results, and discussion (IMRAD) structure: A fifty-year survey. *Journal of the Medical Library Association, 92*(3), 364–367.

Stetler, C. B., Legro, M. W., Rycroft-Malone, J., Bowman, C., Curran, G., Guihan, M., . . . Wallace, C. M. (2006). Role of "external facilitation" in implementation of research findings: A qualitative evaluation of facilitation experiences in the Veterans Health Administration. *Implementation Science, 1*, 23.

Stringer, M. J., Sales-Pardo, M., & Nunes Amaral, L. A. (2008). Effectiveness of journal ranking schemes as a tool for locating information. *PLoS One, 3*(2), e1683.

Stroup, D. F., Berlin, J. A., Morton, S. C., Olkin, I., Williamson, G. D., Rennie, D., . . . Thacker, S. B. (2000). Meta-analysis of observational studies in epidemiology: A proposal for reporting. Meta-analysis of observational studies in epidemiology (MOOSE) group. *Journal of the American Medical Association, 283*(15), 2008–2012.

Title 45 Code of Federal Regulations Part 46. (1991). *Protection of human subjects.* Available from http://www.hhs.gov/ohrp/humansubjects/guidance/45cfr46.htm.

Toft, C. A., & Jaeger, R. G. (1998). Writing for scientific journals I: The manuscript. *Herpetologica, 54*, S42–S54.

Tufte, E. R. (1983). *The visual display of quantitative information.* Chesshire, CT: Graphics Press.

U.S. Department of Health and Human Services (DHHS), Office of Research Integrity. (1990). *First annual report: Scientific misconduct investigations.* Washington DC: Government Printing Services.

Van Way, C. W., 3rd. (2007). Writing a scientific paper. *Nutrition in Clinical Practice, 22*(6), 636–640.

Vanrooyan, S. (1990). A critical examination of the peer review process. *Learned Publishing, 11*, 185–191.

Wald, C. (2008). Economics: Crazy money. *Science, 12*(322), 1624–1626.

Wasserman, T., Murry, T., Johnson, J. T., & Myers, E. N. (2001). Management of swallowing in supraglottic and extended supraglottic laryngectomy patients. *Head and Neck, 23*(12), 1043–1048.

Webb, C. (2002). How to make your article more readable. *Journal of Advanced Nursing, 38*(1), 1–2.

White, L. J. (2002). Writing for publication in biomedical journals. *Prehospital Emergency Care, 6*(Suppl. 2), S32–S37.

World Medical Association. (2000, October). World Medical Association Declaration of Helsinki: Ethical principles for medical research involving human subjects. Available from http://www.wma.net/e/policy/17-c_e.html, 1–7.

Wright, S. M., & Kouroukis, C. (2000). Capturing zebras: What to do with a reportable case. *Canadian Medial Association Journal, 163*(4), 429–431.

Wuchty, S., Jones, B. F., & Uzzi, B. (2007). The increasing dominance of teams in production of knowledge. *Science, 316*(5827), 1036–1039.

Zeller, A., Ramseier, E., Teagtmeyer, A., & Battegay, E. (2008). Patients' self-reported adherence to cardiovascular medication using electronic monitors as comparators. *Hypertension Research, 31*(11), 2037–2043.

Zeller, A., Schroeder, K., & Peters, T. J. (2007). Electronic pillboxes (MEMS) to assess the relationship between medication adherence and blood pressure control in primary care. *Scandinavian Journal of Primary Health Care, 25*(4), 202–207.

Zeller, A., Schroeder, K., & Peters, T. J. (2008). An adherence self-report questionnaire facilitated the differentiation between nonadherence and nonresponse to antihypertensive treatment. *Journal of Clinical Epidemiology, 61*(3), 282–288.

Zeller, A., Taegtmeyer, A., Martina, B., Battegay, E., & Tschudi, P. (2008). Physicians' ability to predict patients' adherence to antihypertensive medication in primary care. *Hypertension Research, 31*(9), 1765–1771.

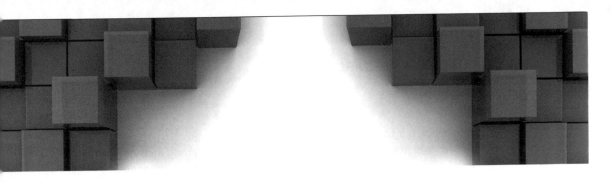

Index